THE POST-
PHYSICIAN ERA _____

HEALTH, MEDICINE, AND SOCIETY:
A WILEY-INTERSCIENCE SERIES

DAVID MECHANIC, Editor

THE POST-
PHYSICIAN ERA_____

Medicine in the Twenty-First Century

JERROLD S. MAXMEN

A WILEY-INTERSCIENCE PUBLICATION

JOHN WILEY & SONS, New York · London · Sydney · Toronto

Library of Congress Cataloging in Publication Data:
Maxmen, Jerrold S.
    The post-physician era.

    "A Wiley-Interscience publication."
    Includes bibliographical references.
    1. Medicine—Philosophy.   2. Medical innova-
tions.   3. Medical personnel.   4. Technological
forecasting.   I. Title.   [DNLM: 1. History of
medicine.   2. Futurology.   WZ40 M464p]

R723M34   610.69'6   76-2442
ISBN 0-471-57880-0

Printed in the United States of America

10 9 8 7 6 5 4 3 2 1

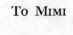
To Mimi

PREFACE

Radical proposals aimed at resolving our health care crisis are presented in this book. I advocate and predict that in the 21st century doctors will be rendered obsolete by a collaboration between the computer and a new breed of health care professional—the medic. Although this proposition flies in the face of popular and academic opinion, I maintain that the emergence of a Post-Physician Era will be feasible, desirable, and inevitable. To support this contention I explore the technological, political, economic, social, and psychohistorical forces that will culminate in the obsolescence of the physician and the establishment of a medic-computer model of health care delivery.

While these developments are occurring, other events will be affecting the future course of medical history. Innovations in communications technology, education, professional roles, biology, and administration will have a profound impact upon the medicine of tomorrow. I examine these areas, especially as they will influence the emergence of a Post-Physician Era.

Although there already are several books in which the future of medicine is discussed, the world of tomorrow is viewed as either an extrapolation or a resurrection of the past. I would suggest that neither perspective is adequate; we cannot solve the problems of the future by resorting to the ineffective policies and programs of the past. Because the future will be unique, its dilemmas will call for new and possibly even unconventional solutions.

The ideas that are advanced here should be of vital concern not only to health care professionals, but also to the general public. Because all of us will be patients at some time in the future, the quality and type of care we will receive may determine if we live and how we live. Decisions about medicine's future are too important to be made by health care professionals alone. Because everyone will be affected by these decisions, ideally everyone should have a voice in determining them. For this participation to occur, however, the public should be fully acquainted with the wide range of options before them. Consequently, this book has been written for a general audience. In doing so I have tried to avoid the use of technical language; whenever such terms were necessary I have tried to explain them.

The advice and expertise of many individuals has been invaluable in preparing this book. I would like to express my appreciation to Edward Sachar, Gary Tucker, and Peter Whybrow for their encouragement and support. I especially would like to extend my gratitude to the National Fund for Medical Education which provided me with a fellowship to research this book. Finally, the secretarial skills of Sue Gregor, Bernice Morton, Jean Ollis, and Nanette Soccino have been instrumental in preparing this manuscript.

JERROLD S. MAXMEN, M.D.

Albert Einstein College of Medicine
Yeshiva University
Bronx, New York
January 1976

CONTENTS

APPENDIX

THE POST-
PHYSICIAN ERA _____

INTRODUCTION

> Doctors are men who prescribe medicine of which they
> know little to cure diseases of which they know less in
> human beings of which they know nothing.

> VOLTAIRE

> The physician strives for the good as the artist strives for
> the beautiful, each pushed on by that admirable feeling we
> call virtue.

> BALZAC

A widespread ambivalence toward the medical profession exists. Some critics fundamentally share Voltaire's cynical attitudes toward physicians. They view doctors as impersonal pseudo-scientists who practice their craft within the confines of an antiquated system in which profits are maximized and health is minimized. More generous souls share Balzac's romanticized perceptions of physicians. They admire the dramatic discoveries of the medical profession and the dedication with which they are

applied. Undoubtedly, these contrasting perspectives have existed as long as has the profession itself. Historically, the prevalence of each of these views has varied, depending upon the
extent to which physicians were believed to have provided, or
have failed to provide, effective and humane treatment. Which of
these attitudes will persist in future generations will be influenced
by the actions of those who plan for the delivery of medical care
in the 21st century.

More than ever before man possesses an interest in planning for
his long-range future. Traditionally, very few individuals seriously considered the distant future; there was no reason to do
so. Because of the slower rate of scientific and cultural change,
man's future life would essentially resemble his present one. Most
likely he would remain in the same village, maintain the same
values, and receive the same medical care. His existence was
characterized by constancy. Today change that once would have
occurred in a generation transpires within a decade (1, 2). Modern
man senses that the accelerating pace of contemporary life will
dramatically alter his future, and thus he has a greater investment
in what that future will bring.

Several developments suggest that our society is increasingly
generating what Harold Lasswell has called "future-oriented
man" (3). In 1966 there was only one college course in futuristics;
by 1974 an estimated 350 to 400 such courses were being
conducted throughout North America (4). During the same
period the membership of the World Future Society had climbed
from zero to 15,000 (5). Scholarly commissions (6, 7) have been
speculating about and planning for life in the year 2000. Numerous journals and publications exclusively concerned with the
future (e.g., *The Futurist, Prevision, Footnotes to the Future,
Futures*) are reaching ever-expanding audiences (5). An active
curiosity about the future is hardly restricted to academics and
futurologists. Books such as *Future Shock* (8), and to a lesser
extent, *The Limits to Growth* (9) and *Profiles of the Future* (10)
have become commercially successful (4). Government officials
are showing a greater interest in technological forecasting as a
way of assessing the consequences of scientific and social innova-

tions (11). Members of professions, such as engineering, economics, and business, are trying to anticipate future developments in their respective fields.

Despite this burgeoning interest in futuristics doctors, who need to be cognizant of prospective medical developments (12–15), have not been inclined to explore the long-range future of medicine Although numerous books have discussed the technical aspects and ethical implications of anticipated biomedical advances, for the most part they have been written by nonphysicians. Medicine certainly entails a great deal more than the biomedical exotica of "test-tube babies," cryogenic preservation, and the like. To most of us, health care primarily means obtaining medical treatment; yet, the topic of how such treatment will be delivered in the *distant* future has received conspicuously little professional or public attention. This book attempts to rectify this deficiency.

WHY EXAMINE MEDICINE'S FUTURE? One could argue that studying the long-range future of medicine—or anything else for that matter—is a waste of time. Considering that we are notoriously unable to predict what will happen in five years, what real benefit is there in seriously attempting to forecast* what will occur over the next half century? For example, the experts once proclaimed that locomotives would never become a popular form of public transportation because their speed of 30 miles per hour would obviously suffocate their passengers (10). As late as 1960 few, if any, of the experts anticipated that in a few years politically moribund college campuses would be transformed into enclaves of militant student radicalism (16). Am I suggesting, therefore, that even the experts consistently fail at prophecy? Precisely. So the question remains: Why bother to examine the future?

Exploring the future can be interesting because we and our

---

* For literary convenience the terms *forecast*, *predict*, and *project* are used interchangeably in this book.

children are going to spend the rest of our lives in it. Other reasons for studying the future are important. By focusing upon specific future developments, one can begin to evaluate their relative desirability. For example, assuming that before 1980 physicians will be able to predict accurately the sex of a child within the first months of pregnancy (17), one can debate and society can decide whether this information should be provided routinely to expectant parents. Undoubtedly, some may argue against this practice, saying that offering this information would diminish the "mystery" of child birth, disrupt the sex balance of the population, and encourage indiscriminate abortion. Conversely, others may view knowing the sex of the fetus as a legitimate parental right and a valuable aid to family planning. Regardless of one's opinion, the point is that by anticipating the potential consequences of a projected development, one is afforded the opportunity to assess its desirability thoroughly *before* the event occurs. Consequently, individuals or society can be better equipped to adopt constructive policies and to avert potential difficulties. Because we are too often unprepared to cope with the consequences of scientific innovations we hastily make decisions that we learn to regret. Studying the future can help to minimize this problem.

Future studies exhibit their greatest utility by projecting alternative futures and by designing policies to accomplish them (15). Dennis Gabor has observed, "The future cannot be predicted, but futures can be invented" (18, p. 175). The futurologist can describe a variety of *alternative futures*. Then we can assess their desirability and probability and determine the best method to obtain what is believed to be the most valuable of them.

Projecting alternative futures is more than a mere intellectual exercise; it has practical consequences. If used judiciously, currently available social and scientific technology can facilitate our efforts to create the future we desire. The medicine of tomorrow does not have to be the result of mysterious and unpredictable forces beyond our control. Instead, we can select the system of health care we want and devise methods to ensure its implementation.

When considering forecasted alternative futures, the reader

should continuously assess the quality of that forecast. Appendix A presents criteria by which the quality of predictions can be evaluated. The presentation of alternative futures in this book include an attempt to answer three distinct, but interrelated questions: (a) What *can* the future be? The answer to this question requires a statement about *feasibility*. (b) What *will* the future be? The answer to this question requires a *predictive* statement. To say that something can occur is quite different from a statement that it will occur. (c) What *should* the future be? The answer to this question requires a *value judgment*. Because something can and will happen does not necessarily mean that it ought to happen. All of these questions must be considered when projecting and evaluating alternative futures.

THREE ALTERNATIVE MEDICAL FUTURES. Although many possibilities could be projected to occur within the next 50 years, throughout this book three different models of health care delivery are focused upon: a physician-centered model, a health-team model, and a medic-computer model. At this point I sketch only their broadest features, leaving more detailed descriptions of them to later. These models are not intended to encompass every aspect of a potential health care system; they focus specifically upon how patients could receive medical care in the future.

Physician-Centered Model. Presently, the dominant model of health care delivery in the United States could be termed a "physician-centered" one. Its primary characteristic is that only the doctor makes diagnostic and treatment decisions. In arriving at diagnostic conclusions the physician may rely upon technological devices, such as electrocardiogram machines or computers, but ultimately the responsibility for rendering these conclusions rests solely with the doctor. Although other health care professionals, such as nurses and social workers, may assist him in executing treatment decisions, the burden of making these decisions falls completely upon the physician. Consequently, patients view the doctor as the central and most critical figure in medical care. All of these characteristics apply to the physician-centered model, whether the doctor practices as a specialist or a generalist, as part of a group or by himself.

Health-Team Model. The majority of diagnostic and treatment tasks in a health-team model would be conducted by allied health professionals.* Physicians would be primarily responsible for coordinating, supervising, and consulting with members of the team and executing highly specialized procedures that paraprofessionals would be unable to perform. Although ultimate clinical and legal responsibility would rest with physicians, in practice most patients would be seen only by allied health personnel. The "doctor-patient" relationship would be superseded by a "paraprofessional-patient" relationship.

To a limited degree the health-team model is already operational. Recently, an increasing number of allied health professionals have been performing routine diagnostic and treatment tasks, which once were considered to be exclusively within the province of the physician. Although this model has been employed most extensively in psychiatry, it also has been utilized in nearly every medical specialty (19).

Medic-Computer Model. A medic-computer model would represent an historically unique method for providing medical services. This third alternative medical future constitutes a radical depar-

---

* In this book the term *allied health professionals* refers to all those individuals, with the exception of physicians, who provide clinical services directly to patients. Although most often they are nurses, social workers, psychologists, and physician's assistants, they also can be members of other occupations. However, not everybody who functions within the health care system is considered to be an allied health professional. For example, because hospital administrators and laboratory technicians do not offer medical care *directly* to patients, they are not referred to as allied health professionals. Throughout this book the terms *allied health professionals*, *allied health personnel*, and *paraprofessionals* are used synonymously.

ture from the other two models. Under this system computers would render most of the technical diagnostic and treatment decisions presently being made by physicians, while *medics*, a hitherto unknown type of health care professional, would provide the supportive and some of the technical tasks currently being performed by doctors. Because a medic-computer symbiosis would usurp all of the tasks presently assigned to physicians, doctors would be rendered obsolete (20). Currently, a medic-computer model would be an impossibility; we do not possess the social or technological resources to create a Post-Physician Era. Nevertheless, as I demonstrate, this model is a feasible, probable, and desirable alternative future.

Ultimately, society will determine which of these three medical alternatives will prevail. Of course, several models may exist concurrently. For example, by the year 2000 ten percent of patients may receive medical care under a physician-centered model, 88 percent under a health-team model, and 2 percent under a medic-computer model. The existence of one model does not preclude the coexistence of another model. During any one time period, however, one system will probably predominate. I would suggest that over the next 50 years this principal model will change more rapidly than at any other time in our history. More specifically, I predict that during the next half century the most prevalent system will evolve from being a physician-centered model to a health-team model and eventually culminate in a medic-computer model.

This revolutionary development will provide patients with both technically and humanistically superior medical care than is being or could *ever* be offered under a physician-centered or a health-team model.

If this hypothesis materializes, it will mean that for the first time in several millennia doctors will cease to exist.

A PERSONAL NOTE. Before proceeding, I feel it is necessary address the issue of why I, a physician, would advocate the obsolescence of doctors, which would mean the termination of my own professional future. Many people have raised questions related to this issue; indeed, I have wondered repeatedly about it myself. Although I firmly believe that the motivations for rendering a proposal should be considered independently of the virtues or the lack of virtues of a proposal *per se*, I feel obliged to explain briefly my primary reason for suggesting the implementation of a Post-Physician Era. I am afraid that by not commenting upon this issue many individuals may fail to examine seriously the merits of a medic-computer model. They might dismiss the entire notion as a product of some hidden ulterior motive of the author. For example, when discussing the concept of a Post-Physician Era before various audiences, some people have responded that I must "have it in" for doctors. Others have claimed that the proposal must derive from my own professional dissatisfactions. Still others have maintained that I am simply enraptured by technology. None of these assertions is correct.

Throughout this book I concentrate on the inherent limitations of the practicing doctor. This focus has been adopted only to demonstrate the necessity of establishing a medic-computer model and *not* to embarrass the medical profession. As a physician and as a patient I have encountered many excellent, thoughtful, and compassionate doctors. My proposal that physicians become obsolete does not stem from any personal dislike for doctors. I believe that physicians have all the virtues and frailties of all humans.

Because there is an intimate relationship between an author and his writings, * I believe it is reasonable to inquire if my desire to see the emergence of a Post-Physician Era derives from some personal professional dissatisfactions. This is not the case. As an academic clinical psychiatrist, my career has been both emotionally satisfying and intellectually rewarding. This is not to say, however, that my professional experiences have not had a significant effect upon the ideas presented in this book. My daily encounters with physicians and allied health personnel have

---

* A favorite teacher of mine was fond of saying that "research is mesearch."

afforded me the opportunity to evaluate their clinical strengths and liabilities. Certainly, these observations have influenced my attitude toward the viability of a medic-computer model.

At first glance one might think that a person who advocates that a machine should usurp the technical decision making functions of the doctor must be a computer zealot. Although I am interested in the medical applications of the machine, this appreciation of its potential clinical uses did not come easily to me. For many years the prospect of an expanding technological society offended my leftist sensitivities. Even today the inner workings of the computer bore me. What I do find intriguing is how the computer can be applied toward the resolution of medical problems and the psychosocial consequences of this application. Furthermore, although I maintain that the computer should play a much greater role in medicine, in no way do I believe that the machine can or should be used to rectify all societal problems. I would like to think that my former technophobic orientation has been superseded by a more dispassionate attitude based on recognition of both the abilities and the liabilities of the machine.

By proposing the eventual replacement of a physician-centered model by a medic-computer model, I hope to present an innovative, viable, and desirable alternative solution to the American health care crisis. Our rapidly changing society is continuously presenting us with new problems, and we must contend with these problems by steadfastly seeking and considering new remedies instead of simply relying on outmoded or all-too-often repeated ideas. The vast majority of proposals aimed at correcting the deficiencies of our medical system have attempted to rearrange the parts of the system without actively questioning the assumptions on which it is based. By challenging the myth of physician necessity I want to explore beyond conventional proposals (e.g., increasing the number of doctors, altering their distribution, or changing their monetary practices). I trust that this book will offer a fresh approach to alleviating the health care dilemmas of tomorrow.

LIMITATIONS ASSUMPTIONS, AND SCOPE.   Any or all of
the forecasts I render in this book may prove to be wrong. Making
long-range projections has always been a risky undertaking.
Witch doctors were imprisoned and burned at the stake for issuing
inaccurate and unpopular predictions. Although modern-day forecasters will not suffer similar penalties, these ancient prophets
share with their 20th-century counterparts the danger of grossly
misjudging the course of future events. For example, in 1926
Edward Bellamy thought that by the year 2000 everyone would
enjoy "magnificent health" (21, p. 222). The projections I am
about to make could turn out to be as inaccurate as Bellamy's prediction. The history of forecasting reveals that more often than
not speculations about the future have proven to be incorrect (10,
22, 23). Why is this?

In making predictions many forecasters have failed to consider
many of the factors that can enhance the quality of a forecast
(see Appendix A). At other times their estimates have been based
upon incorrect or incomplete data. Furthermore, while some forecasters appear to lack imagination (24), others actually seem to
fear it. Arthur Clarke believes the later tendency is more prevalent and refers to it as "failures of nerve" (10, p. 1), which occur
when even though all of the necessary facts are available, the
would-be prophet cannot see that they point to an inescapable
conclusion. Throughout history almost every significant innovative idea has been greeted with a statement such as, "It can't be
done." Clarke cites the example of the great American astrono-
mer Simon Newcomb, who was clever enough to envision that if
gravity could be neutralized, air flight would become possible.
Yet, upon hearing of the Wright brothers' success, he replied that
although flying machines might be a remote possibility, they certainly could not support the weight of anyone besides a pilot.
Newcomb did not lack imagination; he feared it (10). This unwillingness to accept the inevitable consequences of available facts is
what so often leads to excessively conservative forecasts.

Another major obstacle that has traditionally plagued forecasters is their inability to anticipate unexpected developments.

Herman Kahn and Anthony Wiener distinguished between synergistic and serendipitous speculations. The former refers to cooperative and interactive events extrapolated from *presently known* facts. Most projections are of this variety; they are limited to conjectures of improvements upon and combinations of currently available knowledge. Serendipity refers to *unexpected* discoveries and applications that futurologists would be unlikely to anticipate (25). Many of these begin as accidents. The X-ray came from a metal key mistakenly being placed upon a film. Penicillin resulted when a breeze blew mold through a laboratory window onto a fortuitously open culture medium (26). An individual living at the beginning of the 19th century would have been unlikely to predict these discoveries, yet they revolutionized medical care. Because serendipitous events are inevitable, they consistently invalidate even the most carefully reasoned projections.

Thomas Kuhn's theories about the history of science provide another clue as to why so many long-range predictions prove to be wrong. He argues that scientific knowledge is not cumulative; it collapses and is rebuilt after every major conceptual shift. *Paradigms* is the term he uses for these overreaching models and theories by which each new scientific era conducts its routine operations (27). Futurologists function under the paradigms of their era, and they attempt to predict events of a distant period— a period that may operate under completely different paradigms. A perennial hazard in making projections is that the paradigms of the present may not necessarily be the paradigms of the future. Although more theoretical and global in his approach, Kuhn's argument is consistent with that of Kahn and Wiener: The emergence of a new paradigm is a serendipitous development.

Although the predictions I set forth are susceptible to all of these difficulties, this fact does not invalidate the primary objective of this book: To demonstrate the feasibility, desirability, and inevitability of a Post-Physician Era.

In rendering projections I have made the following assumptions: Civilization will not be annihilated by warfare, pestilence, or ecological disasters. A population explosion or a shortage of food and housing will not result in a decreased standard of living for those who inhabit the more industrialized nations. There will be a generally stable or even a gradually improving global economic climate. Technologically advanced countries will not undergo a major cultural transformation, such as that portrayed in Charles Reich's *Greening of America* (28). Receiving good medical care will be valued by the citizenry. Natural resources will be in sufficient supply to allow for continued technological growth. Although these events and trends may not occur, a full exploration of their probability would be beyond the scope of this book.

To prevent this book from becoming unwieldy I focus only upon selected aspects of medicine's future; how health care could be delivered, who could provide it, and how they could be trained. I attend primarily to the rationale for and the operations of a medic-computer model. Other topics, such as future patterns of disease and its treatment, anticipated developments in biomedical communications, and the "New Biology" and its ethical implications are discussed, especially as they relate to medical practice in a Post-Physician Era. My speculations are limited to the health care system as it may exist in the more economically developed countries within the next 50 years. By circumscribing the province of this book to these subjects, I do not wish to denigrate the importance of other topics, such as the economics of health care, potential therapeutic innovations, and anticipated global health issues. But I am reminded of Raymond Bauer's observation:

> The problem is akin to that of how one can eat an elephant. The only answer is that one might begin by biting the elephant. And, considering the magnitude of the task, it is difficult to argue that one place is better than another for biting to start. And, after a considerable amount of biting has taken place, the elephant remains largely unscathed (29, p. 240).

Nevertheless, one has to start some place.

NOTES

1. Lifton, R. J. (1971). "Protean Man." In *History and Human Survival: Essays on the Young and Old, Survivors and the Dead, Peace and War, and on Contemporary Psychohistory*. New York: Vintage. Pp. 311–331.

2. Keniston, K. (1971). "The Speed-up of Change." In *Youth and Dissent: The Rise of A New Opposition*. New York: Harcourt Brace Jovanovich. Pp. 58–80.

3. Lasswell, H. D. (1966). "Future-oriented Man." *American Journal of Psychoanalysis*, 26:157–168.

4. Rojas, B., and H. W. Eldredge (1974). "Status Report: Sample Syllabi and Directory of Futures Studies.' In A. Toffler (ed.), *Learning for Tomorrow: The Role of the Future in Education*. New York: Vintage. Pp. 345–399.

5. *The Futurist* (1974). "Statistical Summary of the World Future Society," 8:90.

6. American Academy of Arts and Sciences (1967). *Toward the Year 2000: Work in Progress. Daedalus*, 96(3).

7. American Academy of Political and Social Science (1973). *The Future Society: Aspects of America in the Year 2000. The Annals*, 408.

8. Toffler, A. (1971). *Future Shock*. New York: Bantam.

9. Meadows, D. H., D. L.Meadows, J. Randers, and W. W. Behrens III (1972). *The Limits to Growth: A Report for the Club of Rome's Project on the Predicament of Mankind*. New York: Universe.

10. Clarke, A. C. (1972). *Profiles of the Future: An Inquiry into the Limits of the Possible*. New York: Bantam.

11. Taviss, I. (1971). "Problems in the Social Control of Biomedical Science and Technology.' In E.Mendelsohn, J. P. Swazey, and I. Taviss (eds.), *Human Aspects of Biomedical Innovation*. Cambridge: Harvard University Press. Pp. 3–45.

12. Schwartz, W. B. (1970). "Medicine and the Computer: The Promise and Problems of Change." *New England Journal of Medicine*, 283:1257–1264.

13. Braunwald, E. (1972). "Future Shock in Academic Medicine." *New England Journal of Medicine*, 286:1031–1035.

14. Maxmen, J. S. (1975). "Forecasting and Medical Education." *Journal of Medical Education*, 50:54–65.

15. McLaughlin, C. P., and A. Sheldon (1974). *The Future and Medical Care: A Health Manager's Guide to Forecasting*. Cambridge: Ballinger.

16. Keniston, K. (1971). *Youth and Dissent: The Rise of A New Opposition*. New York: Harcourt Brace Jovanovich.

17. Gordon, T. J., and R. H. Ament (1969). *Forecasts of Some Technological and Scientific Developments and Their Societal Consequences.* Middletown, Conn.: Institute for the Future, Number R-6.

18. Gabor, D. (1964). *Inventing the Future*. New York: Knopf.

19. Sadler, A.M., Jr., B. L. Sadler, and A. A. Bliss (1972). *The Physician's Assistant: Today and Tomorrow*. New Haven: Yale University Press.

20. Maxmen, J. S. (1973). "Goodbye, Dr. Welby." *Social Policy*, 3(4 & 5):97–106.

21. Bellamy, E. (1926). *Looking Backward 2000–1887*. Boston: Houghton Mifflin.

22. Kiefer, D. M. (1971). "Assessing Technology Assessment." *The Futurist*, 5:234–239.

23. Martino, J. (1968). "Blunders of Negative Forecasting." *The Futurist*, 2:120.

24. Amara, R. C., and G. R. Salancik (1972). "Forecasting: From Conjectural Art Toward Science." *The Futurist*, 6:112–117.

25. Kahn, H., and A. J. Wiener (1967). *Toward the Year 2000: A Framework for Speculation*. New York: Macmillan.

26. Fletcher, J. (1974). *The Ethics of Genetic Control: Ending Reproductive Roulette*. Garden City, N.J.: Anchor.

27. Kuhn, T. S. (1971). *The Structure of Scientific Revolutions*. Chicago: University of Chicago Press.

28. Reich, C. A. (1970). *The Greening of America: How the Youth Revolution Is Trying to Make America Livable*. New York: Random House.

29. Bauer, R. (1971). *The Futurist*, 5:240.

1

THE DEMISE
OF THE PHYSICIAN⎯⎯⎯⎯⎯⎯⎯

We are entering into a new medical era—an era I believe will culminate in the total obsolescence of the physician and in a radical transformation of our entire health care system. The medicine of tomorrow will be significantly different from the medicine of today. The past 75 years of medical history have been characterized by unprecedented change. The introduction of potent therapeutic measures, the rapidly expanding involvement of governments in the delivery of health care, the major reorganization of American medical education, the growth of specialization, and the emergence of a predominately scientific orientation to the practice of medicine—all suggest that change has been the only constant.

Medical history will undoubtedly continue to undergo important, even revolutionary, modifications. From an historical perspective I maintain that the most revolutionary of these changes will be the gradual demise of the physician. This projection is based upon an assessment of the role that allied health professionals and computer technology can and will play in providing medical care as well as an analysis of the specific tasks doctors presently conduct. I attempt to show that in the future all of the functions currently performed by physicians can be accomplished by a partnership of paraprofessionals and computers. As I document this conclusion, the reader will undoubtedly think of a number of technical, philosophical, ethical, economic, and psychological questions about the feasibility, inevitability, or desirability of physicians becoming obsolete. These questions are not to be minimized; they are of critical importance in determining whether a medic-computer will be a viable and humane alternative future. For the sake of clarity, however, I will discuss these issues in the following chapter.

THE TASKS OF THE PHYSICIAN.   The contemporary doctor performs a variety of functions that can be divided into clinical and nonclinical endeavors (see Table 1). According to the American Medical Association, at the end of 1973 physicians in the United States devoted 80.6 percent of their time to patient care, 3.3 percent to administration, 2.3 percent to research, 1.7 percent to education, and 0.7 percent to other unspecified activities. The remaining 11.5 percent of physicians' time could not be ascertained or was spent in retirement (1). Because 91 percent of the time of surveyed working doctors is expended in the clinical sphere, the performance of these activities constitutes the major rationale for the continued existence of the medical profession. Nevertheless, *all* of these tasks could be conducted either by computers or by a new class of health care professionals whom I call "medics."

CLINICAL ACTIVITIES
Disease-Centered Activities.   A physician diagnoses and treats illness by following a standardized routine. He (*a*) takes a history, (*b*) conducts a physical examination, and (*c*) orders ancillary tests. On the basis of these three sources of information, he (*d*) formulates a diagnosis and (*e*) institutes treatment. Upon considering

TABLE I. FUNCTIONS OF THE CONTEMPORARY PHYSICIAN

I. Clinical
    A. Disease-centered Activities
        1. History taking
        2. Physical examination
        3. Ancillary tests
        4. Diagnosis
        5. Treatment
            a. Medication
            b. Psychotherapy
            c. Surgery
        6. Prognosis
    B. Supportive Activities
        1. Emotional
        2. Educative
        3. Integrative
    C. Preventive Health Activities
        1. Patient health measures
            a. Periodic health examinations
            b. Prophylactic treatments
        2. Public health measures
II. Nonclinical
    A. Research
    B. Education
    C. Administration
        1. Patient
        2. Organizational

both the patient's diagnosis and his response to treatment, the doctor (f) renders a prognosis. Various trends would suggest, however, that in the future these six activities need not be performed by a physician.

History Taking.   When gathering a history the physician asks an extensive series of questions about the patient's demographic status, current symptoms, past illnesses, personal habits, emotional state, familial diseases, and so on. These inquiries help him determine the particular illness or illnesses that afflict the patient from among numerable possibilities. The doctor intuitively employs a type of "branching" logic—that is, the questions he asks are partially determined by the previous responses of the patient. For example, if the patient denies having abdominal pain, the doctor will ask about something else; but if the patient indicates that he does have abdominal pain, the physician will inquire further into the nature of this complaint. He may ask how long the symptom has been present, if it becomes aggravated when moving, and so on. The information derived from these questions helps him to determine the proper diagnosis. Although history taking is an invaluable part of clinical medicine, it does not necessarily need to be performed by a physician.

Computers have already been utilized to gather medical histories (2–8). One typical system (3) employs a high-speed digital computer equipped with on-line and real-time processing.* The patient sits before a cathode ray tube and a typewriter keyboard, which enters information directly into the processing unit of the computer. Initially the cathode ray tube, which looks like a television screen, provides instructions for the patient on how to use the system. After offering a few words of encouragement, the machine begins to take a history by displaying a series of questions. Each question is accompanied by a set of answers from which the patient selects one and types it on the keyboard. Subsequent inquiries are made depending upon the answers given by the patient. In this manner the computer utilizes a form of branching logic, which is more systematic and rational than that used by the physician. Because the computer's questions are tailored to the particular problems of the patient, the machine does not waste time asking irrelevant questions.

Many refinements and improvements of this basic system are in use. Rather than typing responses on a keyboard, others have found it easier for patients to touch their finger or point with a pen light to the correct answer on the cathode ray tube (4, 9). Some automated history takers are programmed so that questions and answers are displayed in both English and Spanish (10).

---

* *On-line processing* refers to collecting information directly by the computer. *Real-time processing* refers to processing data as fast as they are generated.

Another important development is a computer that modifies its clinical interview in response to certain nonverbal activities of the patient, such as his heart rate and response latency (the time between the display of a question on the screen and his reply to it on the keyboard). A heart rate that increases significantly after a particular question has been asked suggests that the inquiry has raised the patient's level of anxiety. On the basis of this information the computer can then alter its interview, depending upon the circumstances. For example, an accelerated heart rate in a cardiac patient may induce the computer to branch to a frame that reads, "Relax, you're doing fine." If the heart rate continues to increase, the machine may turn to a less anxiety-provoking subject. Later, when the patient is calmer, the machine can return to the unsettling question. However, if during a *psychiatric* interview a specific inquiry increases the patient's heart rate, the computer could explore the topic in greater depth. A prolonged response latency (greater, for example, than 15 seconds) may indicate that the patient is having some kind of difficulty answering the question. The computer can ask the patient if he would prefer to have the question reworded, clarified, or skipped. An extended response latency to many questions may signal that the patient is either inattentive or has a depressed sensorium. In these situations a paraprofessional could assist the patient in responding to the automated inquiries (11). Already nurses and physician's assistants have been trained to perform this task (12–14).

In the near future automated histories may be taken without the patient being present before a computer. A patient can press the appropriate pushbutton on a Touch-Tone telephone in response to questions being generated orally from a central computer console (15). The verbal questions emanating from the machine are prerecorded, and they, like the visual displays on the cathode ray tube, branch, depending upon the patient's answers. In the more distant future computers will be able to participate in a verbal dialogue with the patient (16–17). Then neither cathode ray tubes nor typewriter keyboards will be necessary to conduct a medical interview.

Computerized history takers have shown their clinical value. Studies have demonstrated that these systems gather histories that are more complete and accurate than those collected by physicians (3, 4, 7, 18–20). Unlike the frequently unintelligible handwritten notes of a doctor, the computer generates a highly legible printout of the patient's medical history (3, 4, 6, 19). The value of a readable patient record should not be underestimated. Because the population is becoming increasingly mobile and because patients are seeing a greater number of specialists, medical records must be legible to many practitioners. Furthermore, the computer's superior capacity to retrieve and transmit patient records (3, 6, 19, 21–23) becomes especially important in emergency room settings where the rapid access to such information can save a life (5). Finally, for purposes of medical audit and research, automated medical histories are preferable to those gathered by physicians (19, 24).

Although the issue of patients' acceptance of the computer will be discussed extensively in the following chapter, here we should note that patients generally have approved of their encounters with automated history taking systems (2–7, 11, 19, 25–26).

Physical Examination.   When conducting a physical examination a doctor attempts to detect unusual enlargements or configurations of organs and to discover any abnormalities in the patient's cardiovascular, pulmonary, nervous and other systems. He utilizes his sense of observation and touch and at times augments these senses by the use of simple instruments, such as a stethoscope, blood pressure cuff, or reflex hammer. Historically, physical examinations were of vital importance in the diagnostic process, and physicians took a great deal of pride in their ability to perform them (27).

Nevertheless, these procedures are being conducted by health professionals other than doctors. Physical examinations performed by nurse-practitioners, nurse-clinicians, and physician's assistants compare favorably to those executed by physicians (12). The results of these examinations have been communicated on-line to the computer and incorporated automatically into the patient's record (12, 22, 28–29).

Despite the historical importance of the physical examination, its significance appears to be on the decline. Information once derived from the physical examination increasingly is being supplied by more sophisticated ancillary tests (30). This trend is disheartening to many older practitioners who prefer to depend upon their own skills rather than to rely upon more complex technological determinations (27). The fact is, however, that when compared to the more accurate clinical methods currently available, the physical examination is notoriously unreliable (21). For example, a phonocardiograph (an instrument for recording heart sounds) is considerably more sensitive and reliable than a stethoscope (31). Furthermore, unlike the stethoscope, the phono-cardiograph can yield a permanent written tracing, which then can be analyzed by a computer (32). The increasing availability of highly accurate and sophisticated diagnostic techniques, such as electrocardiography (EKGs), electroencephalography (EEGs), organ scanning,* tomography,† ultrasound,‡ thermography,§ are gradually rendering the physical examination obsolete.

* Organ scanning is a technique that enables the practitioner to determine the size, configuration, and the existence of some types of pathological changes in certain organs, such as the brain, heart, and thyroid gland. Because many diseased organs pick up radioactive isotopes differently than do normal ones, a device similar to a Geiger counter can be used to show the abnormal patterns by which these affected organs emit electrons. A radiation map can be produced which often helps the doctor spot illnesses that otherwise would go undetected in a physical examination.

† Tomography is an X-ray technique by which detailed images of structures lying in a predetermined plane of tissue can be identified by blurring or eliminating images of structures in the surrounding planes.

‡ Ultrasound involves the use of an electronic device that detects the echoes of inaudible high frequency sound waves as they bounce off organs, bones, and other tissues. Among other things, ultrasonics can be used to determine the size and position of a fetus without causing any harm or discomfort to the mother.

§ Thermography is a procedure that capitalizes upon the fact that heat emanating from a particular part of the body may indicate the presence on inflammation or cancer. Because heat eventually can be converted into light, a special camera can be used to produce a photograph of the diseased area of the body. This photograph can depict minute temperature changes that would not be detectable by a physical examination.

Laboratory tests and X-rays are becoming so widely used that many physicians are making diagnoses primarily upon the results of these determinations. In one study a group of experienced physicians were asked how they would diagnose a patient who complained of chest pain. The doctors were free to ask any questions they desired. In reaching the correct conclusion the two most significant questions were not what the results of the history and physical examination were, but rather what the chest X-ray and EKG showed (33). This study indicates that for investigating the cause of chest pain, the history and physical examination were of less diagnostic value than were the EKG and chest film. One might argue that this study confirms the belief that contemporary doctors have lost the art of knowing how to conduct a good history and physical exam because they rely excessively upon technology. Such a conclusion would be unwarranted. These physicians were highly knowledgeable practitioners, perfectly capable of asking the proper clinical questions. The deficiency in reaching the correct diagnosis lies *not* in the doctor's talents, but in the relatively limited capacity of the history and physical exam to make the proper assessment, regardless of how well they are performed. By the 21st century blood pressure cuffs and stethoscopes may become museum pieces, and the physical examination may be retired to its respected place in medical history.

Ancillary Tests.   Ancillary tests include a wide assortment of diagnostic procedures such as laboratory studies (e.g., blood counts, urinalyses, liver function tests), X-rays, EKGs, and EEGs. In former times these tests were truly "ancillary"—that is, they were a source of information which *supplemented* the data obtained from the history and the physical examination. As a result of technological advances, however, these tests have become increasingly sophisticated, accurate, inexpensive, and available. The large amounts of information that accrue from these procedures are rapidly becoming the single most valuable source of data in the diagnostic process.

The clinical use of ancillary tests occurs in three stages: They are ordered, performed, and interpreted. All three of these tasks can be performed without a doctor. Presently the physician utilizes the information derived from the history and the physical examination to determine which ancillary tests will assist him in reaching a diagnosis. Computers already have been programmed to select these tests based upon the results of the history and the physical examination (22, 34–36). Ancillary tests are routinely conducted by paramedical personnel, such as X-ray and laboratory technicians. The introduction of automated clinical laboratories has raised the efficiency and lowered the costs of performing many of these procedures. Furthermore, the results from these automated laboratories can be transmitted rapidly to the patient's chart in a highly legible and retrievable form (22, 37–39).

The interpretation of ancillary tests is the most vital step in the application of these auxillary procedures. Until recently some of these tests, such as EKGs and X-rays, could have been analyzed only by a doctor. Technology also is rapidly usurping this task of the physician. Computers have been developed that accurately interpret EKGs, as well as if not better than doctors (13, 24, 32, 40–42). Many physicians lack the knowledge or the experience to analyze correctly the many complex patterns of the EKG. Errors are committed not only by the inexperienced or the inadequately trained practitioner; an expert cardiologist can also misdiagnose an EKG. Maintaining a consistently high level of precision is extremely difficult for even the best electrocardiographer, considering the numerous EKGs he is required to read (43). Inevitably, tedium sets in. It is no wonder, therefore, that the use of automated EKGs has recently mushroomed. In 1973 there were nearly 50 commercial firms that marketed these computerized systems in the United States alone. They have been used extensively in large city hospitals where the ever-increasing volume of EKG tracings is overburdening the relatively fixed supply of qualified electrocardiographers. Automated EKGs have also been of inordinate value to people in rural areas, which do not have such highly trained individuals (44).

Whether a doctor works in the city or in the country, has a large or a small practice, a high-quality EKG interpretation is as close as the nearest telephone. With the Phone-A-Gram system, for example, the physician simply inserts one end of a cable into a transmitter and places the other end of it onto the patient's limbs and chest. He dials the Phone-A-Gram computer center, and after giving the center's operator the patient's vital statistics, the doctor places his phone on the transmitter and pushes the start button. Electrical signals emanating from the patient are sent via the transmitter, through conventional telephone wires, to the computer. Within minutes the computer analyzes the EKG. The interpretation is then read to the clinician by the operator, who also immediately mails him a copy of it (45).

The cost of performing and interpreting a typical EKG is $25 to $35, but automated readings can be provided for only $15. Because the use of computerized EKGs saves both time and money without sacrificing quality, forecasters suggest that by 1980 more than 100 million computer-assisted EKGs will be taken annually (46).

By using an analog-to-digital converter (a device that turns a continuous electric voltage into a discrete digital form), not only EKGs, but continuous readings of EEGs, blood pressures, temperatures, chemical analyses, and so on can be performed by a computer (13, 32, 47). Optical scanning techniques also have been developed that can reliably interpret X-rays (13, 24, 41, 48), chromosome (24, 32, 48), blood (48–49), and Pap smears (13). Although the sophisticated equipment needed to choose, perform, and interpret ancillary tests is not yet widely available, it has been developed. As a result, the use of ancillary tests could be conducted in the future without a doctor.

Diagnosis. Based upon the findings of the history, physical examination, and ancillary tests, the physician makes a tentative diagnosis of the patient's condition. This diagnosis is reached intuitively from his knowledge that a certain disorder would be the most likely one for that particular patient, given his signs, symptoms, age, sex, race, and so on. Because a diagnosis involves the use of probabilities, the doctor's intuitively derived conclusions can be expressed in terms of more rigorous mathematical formulas. Correctly programmed computers can utilize these formulas to reach a diagnostic determination (32, 50–51).

Computers have already been devised that accurately diagnose a wide range of illnesses, including congenital (48, 52–54) and rheumatic heart diseases (48), neurological disorders (51, 55), bone (56) and lung tumors (50), acid-base problems (36), Cushing's syndrome (57), arthritic disorders (58), pelvic conditions (59), thyroid abnormalities (60–61), ulcers (62), and psychiatric diseases (7, 63–68).

Although a computer-rendered diagnosis of psychiatric disorders is usually accomplished by analyzing the patient's signs and symptoms, a recently developed technique offers an intriguing alternative method for diagnosing at least some mental illnesses. A commonly recognized behavioral characteristic of schizophrenic patients is their frequent use of bizarre and delusional speech. In many respects their verbal productions closely resemble the dreams of psychiatrically normal individuals. Despite these similarities, Tucker and Rosenberg were able to program a computer to distinguish between transcripts of schizophrenic speech and transcripts of the dream content of normal people. Moreover, their computer was able to differentiate between the recorded language of schizophrenic individuals and the transcribed speech of patients with other psychiatric diagnoses (63). If more extensive research verifies the reliability of their findings and if verbal productions could be automatically transcribed and communicated on-line into the computer, in the future the machine could make a diagnosis of some psychiatric illnesses merely by having the patient speak to the computer.

What is most striking about all of these cybernated methods is that they often diagnose with greater accuracy than can an experienced physician. At present the greatest inhibiting factor to the *widespread* use of automated diagnosis has been our failure to develop sufficient computer facilities, not our technical ability to program these machines. Nevertheless, by the 21st century computers will become as commonplace as television is today

(69–70), and the diagnostic functions of a physician will be usurped totally by the machine.

Treatment. Once the physician has made a diagnosis, he has to choose and implement the most appropriate form of treatment. Like deciding upon the proper diagnosis, determining the course of treatment that will most likely alleviate or cure the patient's illness is a matter of probabilities. Computer systems have been devised to make accurate treatment decisions in the management of severe burns (15), acid-base problems (24, 71), respiratory difficulties (72–73), radiation therapy (74–75), anesthesiology (12), psychiatric illnesses (68, 76), diabetes (77), and cardiac diseases (73).

To determine the proper therapy is one thing; to implement it is quite another. Essentially, contemporary medical treatment consists of any one or a combination of the following: medication, psychotherapy, and surgery. By the 21st century I would suggest that conducting all of these treatment modalities without a physician will be feasible, with one possible minor exception.

Because the treatment of disease usually involves the use of medication, itself a product of technology, the doctor, or more frequently the nurse or pharmacist, simply dispenses the agent that will alleviate the patient's illness. Often the physician is given credit for having cured the patient, when in reality the medication deserves the credit. Benjamin Franklin once observed, "God heals and the doctor takes the fee." Today his dictum could be revised to read, "Drugs heal but the doctor takes the credit." If computers can select the proper medication, what is left for the physician to do? His remaining tasks would consist of monitoring drug side effects and ensuring that patients do not receive contraindicated medications. Computers have been programmed to perform both of these functions (22, 78–79).

Although physicians (usually psychiatrists) do conduct psychotherapy,* one hardly has to be a physician to do so. Nurse-

---

* In this book the term *psychotherapy* refers to a broad range of nonbiological

clinicians, social workers, and especially psychologists have always been among our most talented and imaginative psychotherapists. Nonphysicians, such as Otto Rank, Theodor Reik, Anna Freud, August Aichorn, Kurt Lewin, Carl Rogers, B. F. Skinner, and Virginia Satir, have all made invaluable contributions to the theory and practice of psychotherapy. Although a doctor thoroughly trained in the biological sciences, Sigmund Freud himself staunchly advocated the use of lay analysts (80). *

Although I suspect they will have a limited application, machines have been programmed to conduct a psychotherapeutic dialog (16–17, 68). As the following examples illustrate, their very existence demonstrates the flexibility of the computer.

COMPUTER—How can I help you?
PERSON—I don't know.
COMPUTER— Try to tell me something about it.
PERSON—No.
COMPUTER—Can you elaborate?
PERSON—I am sick and tired today.
COMPUTER—Do you have any idea why?
PERSON—Yes, I'm old.
COMPUTER—Please go on.
PERSON—I seem to have lost interest in everything.
COMPUTER—Tell me more about such feelings.
PERSON—I have some idea why I feel this way too.
COMPUTER—You have?
PERSON—It seems that I miss having a family (16).

Many individuals who have interacted with these psychiatric computers feel annoyed and frustrated with the machine's response. Despite this, the computer seems to take it all in stride.

PERSON—I don't understand.

---

psychological treatment modalities having a multiplicity of orientations, such as psychoanalytic, gestalt, transactional, or behavioral. They may be conducted with an individual, couple, family, or group.
* Lay analysts is the term used for nonphysicians who practice psychoanalysis.

COMPUTER—Do you want to understand?
PERSON—I hate you stupid machine.
COMPUTER—What don't you like about me?
PERSON—You have no feelings.
COMPUTER—How do you mean?
PERSON—I mean you cannot experience what I experience because you are just a machine.
COMPUTER—Tell me more about such feelings.
PERSON—We are not communicating.
COMPUTER—I am trying my best to communicate with you (16).*

The responses of the computer may seem mechanical and stilted and a parody of the psychoanalyst. The style of this dialog *does* approximate the conversation frequently heard in many psychotherapists' offices.

A comparison of the efficacy of computer versus human-conducted psychotherapy is difficult because the usefulness of psychotherapy itself is controversial. Although the majority of clinicians feel that psychotherapy is valuable, a sizable minority do not (81). However, regardless of one's opinion about the value of psychotherapy, it undoubtedly will continue to be practiced in the future. In most circumstances it will be performed by humans, but automated psychotherapy may play a greater role. Once computers are able to conduct a natural verbal dialog they could be linked to conventional telephones, thereby enabling an individual to receive psychotherapy over the phone whenever and for as long as he chooses. The time and duration of the session could fit the needs of the patient, rather than the schedule of the therapist. It also could be more economical than conventional psychotherapy, which often costs between $35 and $50 per hour. A similar amount of computer time costs between $1.50 and $ 4.50, depending upon its availability (7).

* Reprinted by permission of The Williams & Wilkins Co. Colby, K. M., J. B. Watt, and J. P. Gilbert (1966). "A Computer Method of Psychotherapy: Preliminary Communication." *Journal of Nervous and Mental Disease*, 142 : 148–152.

In addition to helping people resolve emotional difficulties, automated psychotherapy may assist individuals in understanding their feelings about the computer. Although people's reactions to the machine are discussed more extensively in the next chapter, at this point we should be aware that such feelings exist and are often expressed with considerable vehemence (82–83). The need to understand these feelings may become of greater importance in the future when our society becomes even more automated. As the above computer-patient transcript illustrates, automated psychotherapy may provide us with an opportunity to confront the machine directly in a very personal, real, and possibly even cathartic manner. Individuals may be able to obtain on an *emotional* level a deeper insight into their attitudes toward the computer as well as a greater appreciation of the machine's powers and limitations. In some respects a dialog with a computer could more readily provide an individual with this understanding than would a conversation with another human.

Regardless of how automated psychotherapy may be utilized, the extent of its future use is difficult to predict. But even if it is not used, the central point is that psychotherapy can be performed effectively by allied health professionals, and therefore, physicians are not required to conduct it.

The final class of therapeutic interventions consists of those procedures that are conducted by surgeons or surgical subspecialists (e.g., obstetricians, ophthalmologists, urologists). Although their tasks are not limited to performing surgery, this function is what distinguishes them from other medical specialists. Because a high degree of manual dexterity is required to perform an operation, this is the area in which the physician would be least likely to be rendered obsolete by a computer. Furthermore, the medic's limited training (Chapter 7) would not prepare him to conduct *complicated* surgical procedures. But even this fact does not mean that the surgeon will survive eternally, nor that many of his activities could not be assumed by other human or technological resources.

Many forms of *minor* surgery, such as suturing wounds and correcting fractures, currently and routinely are performed by military corpsmen and physician's assistants (84). Although in this country babies generally have been delivered by obstetricians, midwives can often assume this responsibility. In England 80 percent of deliveries are performed by midwives; a majority of births in Sweden, Germany, and Holland also are conducted by midwives (85). Even in the United States the demand for their services has been on the rise. The shortage of doctors, economic considerations, the feminist movement, and the desire of many women to have their babies at home under constant supervision have all led to an increased number of American midwives. Whereas in 1962 there were only 400 certified midwives in the United States, one decade later there were about 5000 (1, 85).

Because the pre- and postoperative functions of a surgeon generally consist of monitoring the patient's physiological processes and, if necessary, correcting them with medication, these functions could be performed by a medic-computer partnership (84, 86). Allied health professionals also have been tranied to execute many of the duties of the anesthesiologist (12, 84). William Schwartz has suggested that if new monitoring techniques were combined with the capacity of the computer to analyze and respond instantaneously to large volumes of physiologic data, the administration of anesthesiology could become a fully automated process (24).

What about *major* surgical intervention? First, many authors claim that in the United States many unnecessary operations are performed (87–91). For example, in comparing equal populations of the United States with England and Wales, about three times more cholecystectomies (excision of the gall bladder), two-and-a-half times more hysterectomies, and two times more inguinal herniorrhaphies and hemorrhoidectomies are conducted in the United States (87). The rate of tonsillectomies in Great Britain is about half that of the United States (90, 91). Lower surgical rates also exist in Sweden (88). Among the reasons advanced to explain the high rate of allegedly unnecessary surgical operations performed in the United States are the fee-for-service payment system (88, 89), the greater degree of solo practice (89), the inadequacy of professional consultation (87, 89–90), and the existence of lesser qualified and more therapeutically aggressive doctors conducting surgery in America (87). Although 1,100,000 tonsillectomies are performed annually in this country, there is considerable competent medical opinion that doubts the long-term efficacy of this procedure. Moreover, these operations cause 200 to 300 deaths per year as well as leading to a sizable amount of infections, hemorrhages, and other serious postoperative sequelae (88, 91). Thus, even though presently there are many legitimate indications for surgical interventions, many operations appear to be harmful as well as unnecessary.

Second, in the future many currently legitimate operations may become unnecessary as further medical discoveries emerge. Many illnesses, such as tuberculosis and ulcers, once thought only to be amenable to surgery, now can be cured largely by the use of medication or diet. Recent advances in the understanding of gallstone formation may obviate the need to remove them surgically within a decade (92). The prenatal administration of effective chemical agents may eliminate the need to operate on many types of congenital abnormalities. Discoveries in embryology, immunology, virology, and biochemistry could result in many disorders being treated in the office, rather than in the operating room. Although the surgical tasks of the physician may be the last ones to be usurped by a medic-computer symbiosis, eventually they too may become obsolete.

Prognosis. The final disease-oriented activity of the doctor consists of offering a prognosis, which is an estimation of the patient's chances of improvement or recovery. These determinations presently are made by the physician based upon his knowledge of the patient's particular disease, the availability of effective treatments, and the patient's response to therapy. As one may surmise, the rendering of a prognosis, just as the making of a diagnosis, is a matter of probabilities, and therefore, readily applicable to computer methods. Already automated systems have been used to provide prognostic determinations (7, 66–67).

In the future the six *technical* disease-oriented tasks of the

physician could be assumed totally by a medic-computer partnership. But contemporary doctors do considerably more than simply
perform technical procedures. They also provide, or at least
should provide, a great deal of *emotional support*. The need for
this support cannot be underestimated; it may prove to be the
critical difference between therapeutic success or failure. Whether
physicians are needed to perform these psychological functions,
however, is quite another matter.

Supportive Activities.   Much of the criticism leveled against contemporary physicians has been over their alleged insensitivity
to their patients' emotional needs. Another closely related complaint is that doctors fail to inform patients about the nature of
their medical problems (93–95). When physicians neglect these
psychological and educational functions, their clients often feel
bewildered and afraid because they neither understand the relative seriousness of their illness nor possess the emotional support
that is necessary to contend optimally with their diseases (95).

Undoubtedly there are many reasons why some physicians do
not provide adequate emotional and educational support for their
patients. Doctors frequently are overworked, preoccupied with
the technical aspects of their jobs, or both. In addition, they tend
to be respected by their colleagues because of their knowledge of
medicine rather than because of their sensitivity to patients. To
acquire this respect, some physicians, especially those in academic
centers, tend to maximize their technical excellence and minimize
emotional support. Unfortunately, these are the doctors who
generally provide the role models from which student-physicians
are expected to learn the humanistic side of patient care. Furthermore, medical students are selected primarily on the basis of their
performance in scientific subjects (96–97) rather than on their
ability to relate to people. Because of the student-physician's
need to acquire a massive amount of scientific information
throughout his training, his formal education tends to augment
his concern with the technical instead of the psychological side of
clinical practice. Although this is a regrettable phenomenon, the

necessity to learn the technical aspects of medicine cannot be underestimated. The acquisition of information is what distinguishes the doctor from the well-intentioned layman.

In the future, however, if most technical activities can be assumed by computers, the medic could focus on providing emotional. support. He would be free to concentrate on the psychological aspects of clinical practice. Unlike the physician, he could be selected primarily on the basis of his interpersonal abilities. Given his innate capacity to empathize and communicate with people, these endowments could be nurtured throughout his formal training (Chapter 7).

Closely related to the supportive functions currently performed by doctors are what I call their "integrative activities." By this term I mean the management of the patient's overall health care. With the growth of medical knowledge, a patient often finds himself shuffled from specialist to specialist, without having any single physician coordinating their efforts (93, 98). Many individuals can say who their doctors are, but not who their doctor is. Many patients do not know to whom they should turn when they require medical care. They seek treatment in hospitals where they see a wide diversity of physicians. Generally speaking, these doctors have neither a long-standing relationship nor a firsthand knowledge of the patient. They must rely upon the patient's medical record for this information. Unfortunately, these records are notoriously disorganized, unintelligible, and unavailable (7, 21, 99). Because there is no adequate source of data, hospital doctors frequently are unable to coordinate a patient's medical care. To resolve this problem some hospitals have established "primary care clinics," in which one physician is assigned permanently to a particular patient. This reorganizational measure, although theoretically desirable, is practically unobtainable. Most hospitals are staffed by interns and residents who usually are affiliated with the institution for only one to three years. Furthermore, they frequently rotate among numerous clinical services to acquire experience in various medical specialties. As a result, they are unable to follow a patient for any sustained period.

Recognizing the lack of coordinated care afforded many

patients, others have suggested the need for a new type of general practitioner, the so-called "family practitioner" (100). This impulse to resurrect the past, however, is doomed to fail. The very forces that led to the demise of the general practitioner (e.g., increased medical knowledge, specialization, decreased status) also will lead to the demise of the family practitioner. One cannot solve a fundamental problem simply by changing someone's title (101). We must look for other solutions.

A medic-computer model could greatly alleviate this dilemma. Because computers eventually will be able to provide the highly technical services of the contemporary specialist, there would be less need for patients to pass from doctor to doctor. The medic would be able to establish a long-standing and enduring relationship with his clients. Because a patient's record would be fully automated, it would be readily accessible and easily comprehended by anyone who had a legitimate need to use it. In addition patients could decide voluntarily to have their medical records contained in a national or even an international medical computer bank (Chapter 3). The increased mobility of the populace, which in part has contributed to the poor integration and continuity of patient care, would no longer be a serious problem.

Preventive Health Activities.   For millennia the importance of preventive health measures has been recognized. As long ago as 2500 B.C. Huang Ti, the Yellow Emperor, said, "The superior physician helps before the early budding of the disease" (102, p. 449). In more recent times the significance of preventive medicine has been more rigorously documented (103–104). Although physicians generally have not focused an inordinate amount of energy in this area, any discussion that is a systematic attempt to demonstrate that a medic-computer model of health care could assume all the tasks of the contemporary physician must include an examination of the doctor's preventive health functions.

A society offers preventive health services to individual patients and the public-at-large. For the most part physicians provide the former activities, while government officials perform the latter.

Those preventive health measures administered to individual patients can be divided further into periodic health examinations * and prophylactic treatment. Although a complete discussion of these topics is beyond the scope of this chapter, I do want to show that these procedures can be carried out in the future without a physician.

Periodic Health Examinations. Possibly the best known comprehensive system for providing patients with periodic health examinations is the Automated Multiphasic Screening Program at the Kaiser-Permanente Health Program in San Franciso-Oakland. Within two to three hours patients receive from allied health professionals an extensive battery of procedures, including a symptom questionnaire, EKG, chest and breast X-rays, tonometry for glaucoma, respirometry for lung diseases, audiometry for hearing deficiencies, and selected blood and urine tests. All of the information derived from these procedures is conveyed to a computer, which can then suggest that further tests be performed (34). In 1969 approximately 500 patients were serviced within a 40-hour week at the relatively low cost of $21.32 per patient (106). The experience of the Kaiser-Permanente Medical Group illustrates that an efficient and economical system can be devised for the administration of screening procedures.† The physician is

* In this book I use the terms *periodic health examination* and *multiphasic screening* interchangeably. Technically speaking, a periodic health examination refers to the application of diagnostic procedures on a regular basis. Multiphasic screening can be defined as the presumptive identification of unrecognized diseases or defects by the utilization of numerous tests, examinations, and procedures that can rapidly distinguish between apparently well persons who probably have a disease from those who probably do not. A screening test is *not* intended to be diagnostic, and individuals with positive or suspicious findings must receive further tests to determine if the person really does have the suspected illness (105). Nevertheless, for simplicity as well as the fact that a periodic health examination usually includes some screening tests, these two terms are used synonymously.

† I do *not* wish to imply that automated screening activities *should* be performed. Instead, I only want to emphasize that although the performance of these procedures is a major task of the contemporary doctor, a physician is not required to conduct them.

involved only to the extent of interpreting X-rays and EKGs, tasks which could, as previously indicated, be performed by a computer.

Prophylactic Treatment. Prophylactic treatments, such as immunizations and vaccinations, are generally prescribed by physicians and executed by nurses. In some clinical settings, however, where physician's assistants and nurses essentially provide all of the "well-baby care," the performance of these tasks routinely include both the prescription and administration of prophylactic treatments. In the future medics or computers could prescribe these procedures and nurses could implement them.

Public Health Measures. To a large extent the health of a nation is a function of the quality of its nutrition, housing, sanitation, and environment (104). For example, in less than a decade the introduction of DDT into Ceylon was largely responsible for a 57 percent decline in the death rate (107). One could reasonably argue that the physical well-being and longevity of a populace is related more closely to the general quality of life within a society than it is to the quality of available medical care.

Unfortunately, medical schools provide neither the instruction nor the encouragement for students to enter public health administration. As a result, doctors have not assumed a major role in the field. Most public health officials have come from professions other than medicine. Graduates of public health schools, city planners, environmental engineers, basic science researchers, and politicians have always, and I suspect, will continue to assume the major responsibility for providing these vital public services. The continued existence of the doctor on the basis of his role in public health cannot be justified.

NONCLINICAL ACTIVITIES.   In recent years the disenchantment with American medicine has been focused largely upon the unavailability of health care services (88, 90, 103, 108). Although this concern is justified, in my opinion it has fostered the beliefs that doctors spend an excessive amount of time performing non-clinical endeavors (e.g., research, training, and administration) and that these endeavors are relatively unimportant. In reality physicians devote less than 10 percent of their time to nonclinical activities (1). Furthermore, the provision of quality medical care depends upon adequate research, training, and administration. Without good research medicine stagnates. Without good training effective medicine cannot be practiced. Without good administration health care delivery becomes chaotic. However, although research, training, and administration are of utmost importance, the continued execution of these vital tasks need not be performed by the physician. Just as his clinical responsibilities could be assumed by medics and computers, his nonclinical activities could be assumed by other allied health personnel and advanced technology.

Research. Medical research has never been within the exclusive province of the doctor. Many significant advances, such as the discovery of penicillin, have been made by the non-physician. Yet one still could argue that the doctor's clinical experience affords him several unique advantages over his non-medical research colleagues. The physician is better able to identify unsolved medical problems and is more likely to understand and apply basic research findings to clinical situations. Although in theory the knowledge acquired from direct patient contact should enhance the physician's investigatory skills, in reality just the opposite often occurs. During the formative years of his training, when he ought to be learning basic scientific principles and methods, the future physician-investigator is forced to assimilate massive quantities of clinical information. Later his patient care responsibilities distract him from *fully* developing and utilizing his investigatory talents. Thus, although the physician-investigator's clinical experience affords him a valuable research perspective, it paradoxically inhibits him from putting this perspective to use.

The nonphysician-investigator is adept scientifically but naive clinically; the physician-investigator is unsophisticated scientifically but experienced clinically. In the future it would be unnecessary to train doctors to become researchers if the nonphysician-investigator could be sensitized to relevant clinical issues (109–110) (see Chapters 5 and 7).

An alternative possibility is that under a medic-computer model the doctor's role could change from clinician to researcher. His training would be modified to emphasize scientific principles and techniques, and the clinical information he acquires would prepare him to conduct medical investigations rather than to perform patient care services. An individual who would receive such an education may still be called a "physician." *Nevertheless, to assign him this label would distort significantly the generally accepted meaning of the term, which is a legally sanctioned practitioner who diagnoses and treats human illnesses.* Under a medic-computer model there may be people known as "physicians," but in reality they would function quite differently from those who currently hold this title. For this reason I believe the phrase "Post-Physician Era" would be an accurate description of the period in which a medic-computer model would become the prevailing mode of health care delivery.

Education. The primary reason we now train physicians is so that they can provide medical care. If eventually the clinical activities of the doctor are rendered obsolete by a medic-computer partnership, the current rationale for educating physicians would cease to exist. Medics could be taught by other medics, just as nurses are taught by other nurses. The advent of a Post-Physician Era would divest the doctor of his traditional educational responsibilities.

Administration. Whether they like it or not, all contemporary doctors assume administrative tasks. These duties can be divided into patient and organizational administration. The former includes a wide assortment of paper work, such as filling out insurance, employee, or school health forms. Most physicians view these responsibilities as necessary evils that accompany clinical practice. In the future even allied health professionals could be freed of the drudgery of having to contend with these exceedingly boring tasks. Because machines will store all medical information, they could generate all required health forms. Already computers have been used to perform these tasks (22–23, 111).

The organizational tasks of the physician consist of an even wider variety of activities, ranging from collecting and distributing laboratory test data to administrating hospitals and medical schools. To perform these duties doctors increasingly are relying upon technology (112). For example, the MIS-1 (Medical Information System) handles all inpatient, outpatient, and emergency room transactions. This includes medical orders, specimen pickup lists, patient care plans, laboratory test results, radiology reports, all drug prescriptions including preparation of pharmacy labels, patient bills, census reports, discharge summaries, and other varied tasks. This system could save a hospital approximately $63,400 per month for the first five years of operation. It would also result in other cost effective improvements, because it would lead to reduced patient stays and more efficient use of ancillary services (113). New York City's Health Services Administration currently uses a computerized screening of insurance claims, which has yielded a savings of between $4.5 and $6 million annually (114). Although experts are not unanimous in their belief that automated information systems will be more economical, most of them do feel that they will lead to the more efficient use of health care personnel (115). As the costs of hospital and medical information systems decrease and as the computer becomes a more integral part of clinical practice, automated techniques undoubtedly will usurp a large portion of the physician's administrative responsibilities.

The use of computerized information systems also can assist administrators in gathering the data necessary for rendering appropriate management decisions (115–116). Ultimately, however, organizational responsibilities will rest with man, not machine. Unfortunately, physicians who have often devoted their lives to the acquisition of clinical skills are unprepared to assume major administrative duties. They generally lack a knowledge of economics, politics, group dynamics, and management skills. In the future schools could be established with a curriculum that integrates the organizational skills of the businessman with the humanitarian orientation of the physician. Its graduates would undoubtedly be better equipped than contemporary doctors to perform these administrative functions (see Chapter 7).

Having systematically reviewed all of the tasks currently performed by the doctor, I have tried to demonstrate the possibility that physicians can be rendered obsolete by a medic-computer symbiosis. At this juncture, however, there not only will be, but ought to be, certain reservations about the feasibility, inevitability, and desirability of a Post-Physician Era. Certainly these questions deserve careful consideration, and therefore, will be examined in the following chapter.

NOTES

1. Eisenberg, B. S., and P. Aherne (eds.) (1974). *Socioeconomic Issues of Health '74*, Chicago: American Medical Association.

2. Coddington, R. D., and T. L. King (1972). "Automated History Taking in Child Psychiatry." *American Journal of Psychiatry*, 129:276–282.

3. Slack, W. V., G. P. Hicks, C. E. Reed, and L. J. Van Cura (1966). "A Computer-Based Medical-History System." *New England Journal of Medicine*, 274:194–198.

4. Mayne, J. G., W. Weksel, and P. N. Sholtz (1968). "Toward Automating the Medical History." *Mayo Clinic Proceedings*, 43(1):1–25.

5. Greist, J. H., L. J. Van Cura, and N. P. Kneppreth (1973). "A Computer Interview for Emergency Room Patients." *Computers and Biomedical Research*, 6:257–265.

6. Greist, J. H., M. H. Klein, and L. J. Van Cura (1973). "A Computer Interview for Psychiatric Patient Target Symptoms." *Archives of General Psychiatry*, 29:247–253.

7. Greist, J. H., D. H. Gustafson, F. F. Stauss, G. L. Rowse, T. P. Laughren,

and J. A. Chiles (1973). "A Computer Interview for Suicide-Risk Prediction." *American Journal of Psychiatry*, 130:1327–1332.

8. Gottlieb, G. L., R. F. Beers, Jr., C. Bernecker, and M. Samter (1972). "An Approach to Automation of Medical Interviews." *Computers and Biomedical Research*, 5:99–107.

9. Weir, R. D. (1968). "The Next Ten Years?" In G. McLachlan and R. A. Shegog (eds.), *Computers in the Service of Medicine: Essays on Current Research and Applications, Volume II*. London: Oxford University Press. Pp. 173–186.

10. Brody, J. E. (1971). "Prevention of Illness Is Aim of New Computerized Testing Here." *New York Times*, March 30. P. 37

11. Slack, W. (1971). "Computer-Based Interviewing System Dealing With Nonverbal Behavior As Well as Keyboard Responses." *Science*, 171(3966): 84–87.

12. Chodoff, P., and C. Gianaris II (1973). "A Nurse-Computer Assisted Preoperative Anesthesia Management System." *Computers and Biomedical Research*, 6:371–392.

13. Payne, L. C. (1969). "The Role of Computers in Medicine." In J. Rose (ed.), *Proceedings of the Symposium on Computers in Medicine*. London: J & A Churchill. Pp. 5–18.

14. Collen, M. F. (1969). "Development of Health Systems-II" In J. F. Dickson III, and J. H. U. Brown (eds.), *Future Goals of Engineering in Biology and Medicine*. New York: Academic Press. Pp. 279–285.

15. Allen, S. I., and M. Otten (1969). "The Telephone As A Computer Imput-Output Terminal for Medical Information." *Journal of the American Medical Association*, 208:673–679.

16. Colby, K. M., J. B. Watt, and J. P. Gilbert (1966). "A Computer Method of Psychotherapy: Preliminary Communication." *Journal of Nervous and Mental Disease*, 142:148–152.

17. Nievergelt, J., and J. C. Farrar (1973). "What Machines Can and Cannot Do." *American Scientist*, 61:309–315.

18. *Psychiatric News* (1973). "Computer Interviews Hailed As Superior to Physicians," 8(6):30.

19. Grossman, J. H., G. O. Barnett, M. T. McGuire, and D. B. Swedlow (1971). "Evaluation of Computer-Acquired Patient Histories." *Journal of the American Medical Association*, 215:1286–1291.

20. Greist, J. H. (1973). Personal Communication, April 6.

21. Bennett, A. E., and W. W. Holland (1968). "The Medical Record and the Computer. Part I." In G. McLachlan and R. A. Shegog (eds.), *Computers in the Service of Medicine: Essays on Current Research and Applications, Volume II*. London: Oxford University Press. Pp. 119–128.

22. *Computers and Medicine* (1974). "An Ambulatory Care Information System," 3(5):3.

23. *Computers and Medicine* (1974). "An Ambulatory Care Information System (continued)," 3(6):3.

24. Schwartz, W. B. (1970). "Medicine and the Computer: The Promise and Problems of Change." *New England Journal of Medicine*, 283:1257–1264.

25. Slack, W. V., and C. W. Slack (1972). "Patient-Computer Dialogue." *New England Journal of Medicine*, 286:1304–1309.

26. Haessler, H. A. (1971). "The Interactive, Self-Administered Medical History." In C. Berkley (ed.), *Automated Multiphasic Health Testing*. New York: Engineering Foundation. Pp. 276–286.

27. Bates, B., and J. Mulinare (1970). "Physicians' Use and Opinions of Screening Tests in Ambulatory Practice." *Journal of the American Medical Association*, 214:2173–2180.

28. Kanner, I. F. (1971). "The Programmed Physical Examination With or Without A Computer." *Journal of the American Medical Association*, 215: 1281–1285.

29. Slack, W. V., B. M. Peckham, L. J. Van Cura, and W. F. Carr (1967). "A Computer-Based Physical Examination System." *Journal of the American Medical Association*, 200:224–228.

30. Knapp, S. R. (1973). "Perspectives on Behavioral Technology." *Medical Marketing and Media*, 8(9):15–22.

31. Carlisle, N., and J. Carlisle (1966). *Marvels of Medical Engineering*. London: Oak Tree Press.

32. Ledley, R. S. (1966). "Computer Aids to Medical Diagnosis." *Journal of the American Medical Association*, 196:933–943.

33. Rutstein D. D. (1967). *The Coming Revolution in Medicine*. Cambridge, Mass.: M.I.T. Press.

34. Collen, M. F. (1966). 'Periodic Health Examinations Using An Automated Multitest Laboratory." *Journal of the American Medical Association*, 195:830–833.

35. Gleser, M. A., and M. F. Collen (1972). "Towards Automated Medical Decisions." *Computers and Biomedical Research*, 5:180–189.

36. Goldberg, M., S. B. Green, M. L. Moss, C. B. Marbach, and D. Garfinkel (1973). "Computer-Based Instruction and Diagnosis of Acid-Base Disorders." *Journal of the American Medical Association*, 223:269–275.

37. Whitehead, T. P., J. F. Becker, and M. Peters (1968). "Data Processing in A Clinical Biochemistry Laboratory." In G. McLachlan and R. A. Shegog (eds.), *Computers in the Service of Medicine: Essays on Current Research and Applications, Volume I*. London: Oxford University Press. Pp. 113–134.

38. Jungner, G. (1969). "Automation in Clinical Laboratories-II." In J. F. Dickson III, and J. H. U. Brown (eds.), *Future Goals of Engineering in Biology and Medicine*. New York: Academic Press. Pp. 227–231.

39. *Computers and Medicine* (1974). "Technological Diagnosis Support," 3(3):3.

40. Hu, K., D. B. Francis, G. T. Gau, and R. E. Smith (1973). "Development and Performance of Mayo-IBM Electrocardiographic Computer Analysis Programs (V70)." *Mayo Clinic Proceedings*, 48:260–268.

41. Stehling, K. R. (1972). *Computers and You*. New York: New American Library.

42. *Computers and Medicine* (1974). "Minicomputer Assists in Diagnosis of Heart Disease," 3(3):4.

43. *Medical World News* (1972). "Interpreting ECGs," 13(47):4–5.

44. Pipberger, H. V., and J. Cornfield (1973). "What ECG Computer Program to Choose for Clinical Application: The Need for Consumer Protection." *Circulation*, 47: 918–920.

45. *Computers and Medicine* (1974). "Computerized ECG Analysis Service," 3(3):4–5.

46. *The Computer-Assisted Electrocardiography (CAE) Market*. (1974). New York: Frost and Sullivan, Inc.

47. Weil, M. H., H. Shubin, and D. Stewart (1969). "Patient Monitoring and Intensive Care Units-I." In J. F. Dickson III and J. H. U. Brown (eds.), *Future Goals of Engineering in Biology and Medicine*. New York: Academic Press. Pp. 232–246.

48. Zarnstorff, W. C., W. R. Hendee, and P. L. Carson (eds.) (1972). *Application of Optical Instrumentation in Medicine*. Chicago: Society of Photo-Optical Instrumentation Engineers.

49. Gordon, B. L. (1970). "Regularization and Stylization of Medical Records." *Journal of the American Medical Association*, 212:1502–1507.

50. Boyle, J. A., and J. A. Anderson (1968). "Computer Diagnosis: Clinical Aspects." *British Medical Journal*, 24:224–229.

51. Wortman, P. M. (1972). "Medical Diagnosis: An Information-Processing Approach." *Computers and Biomedical Research*, 5:315–328.

52. Warner, H. R., A. F. Toronto, L. G. Veasey, and R. Stephenson (1961). "A Mathematical Approach to Medical Diagnosis: Application to Congenital Heart Disease." *Journal of the American Medical Association*, **177**: 177–183.

53. Templeton, A. W., J. L. Lehr, and C. Simmons (1966). "The Computer Evaluation and Diagnosis of Congenital Heart Disease, Using Roentgenographic Findings." *Radiology*, 87:658–670.

54. Toronto, A. F., L. G. Veasey, and H. R. Warner (1963). "Evaluation of A Computer Program for Diagnosis of Congenital Heart Disease." *Progress in Cardiovascular Diseases*, 5:362–377.

55. Meyer, A. U., and W. K. Weissman (1973). "Computer Analysis of the Clinical Neurological Examination." *Computers in Biology and Medicine*, 3: 111–117.

56. Lodwick, G. S., C. L. Haun, W. E. Smith, R. F. Keller, and E. E. Robertson (1963). "Computer Diagnosis of Primary Bone Tumors: A Preliminary Report." *Radiology*, 80:273–275.

57. Nugent, C. A., H. R. Warner, J. T. Dunn, and F. H. Tyler (1964). "Probability Theory in the Diagnosis of Cushing's Syndrome." *The Journal of Clinical Endocrinology and Metabolism*, 24:621–627.

58. McGirr, E. M. (1969). "Computers in Clinical Diagnosis." In J. Rose (ed.), *Proceedings of the Symposium on Computers in Medicine.* London: J & A Churchill. Pp. 19–31.

59. Eden, M. (1969). "Computers in Biomedicine-II." In J. F. Dickson III, and J. H. U. Brown (eds.), *Future Goals of Engineering in Biology and Medicine.* New York: Academic Press. Pp. 216–221.

60. Overall, J. E., and C. M. Williams (1963). "Conditional Probability Program for Diagnosis of Thyroid Function." *Journal of the American Medical Association,* 183:307–313.

61. Boyle, J. A., W. R. Greig, D. A. Franklin, R. McG. Harden, W. W. Buchanan, and E. M. McGirr (1966). "Construction of A Model for Computer-Assisted Diagnosis: Application to the Problem of Non-Toxic Goitre." *Quarterly Journal of Medicine,* 35(140):565–588.

62. Wilson, W. J., A. W. Templeton, A. H. Turner, and G. S. Lodwick (1965). "The Computer Analysis and Diagnosis of Gastric Ulcers." *Radiology,* 85: 1064–1073.

63. Tucker, G. J., and S. D. Rosenberg (1975). "Computer Content Analysis of Schizophrenic Speech: A Preliminary Report. *American Journal of Psychiatry,* 132:611–616.

64. Spitzer, R. L., J. Endicott, J. Cohen, and J. L. Fleiss (1974). "Constraints on the Validity of Computer Diagnosis." *Archives of General Psychiatry,* 31: 197–203,

65. Spitzer, R. L., and J. Endicott (1969). 'DIAGNO II: Further Developments in A Computer Program for Psychiatric Diagnosis." *American Journal of Psychiatry,* 125(January Supplement):12–21.

66. Sletten, I. W., H. Altman, and G. A. Ulett (1971). "Routine Diagnosis by Computer." *American Journal of Psychiatry,* 127:1147–1152.

67. Finney, J. C., D. E. Skeeters, C. D. Auvenshine, and D. F. Smith (1973). "Phases of Psychopathology After Assassination." *American Journal of Psychiatry,* 130:1379–1380.

68. American Psychiatric Association (1971). *Automation and Data Processing in Psychiatry.* Task Force Report Number 3. Washington, D. C: American Psychiatric Association.

69. Kemeny, J. G. (1972). *Man and the Computer.* New York: Scribner's.

70. Sarnoff, D. (1966). "No Life Untouched." *Saturday Review,* 49(30): 21–22.

71. Bleich, H. L. (1969). "Computer Evaluation of Acid-Base Disorders." *Journal of Clinical Investigation,* 48:1689–1696.

72. Menn. S. J., G. O. Barnett, D. Schmechel, W. D. Owens, and H. Pontoppidan (1973). "A Computer Program to Assist in the Care of Acute Respiratory Failure." *Journal of the American Medical Association,* 223: 308–312.

73. Warner, H. R., C. M. Olmsted, and B. D. Rutherford (1972). "HELP—A Program for Medical Decision-Making." *Computers and Biomedical Research,* 5(1):65–74.

74. Parr, R. F., and J. A. Newell (1968). "Radiotherapy Treatment Planning." In G. McLachlan, and R. A. Shegog (eds.), *Computers in the Service of Medicine: Essays on Current Research and Application, Volume I.* London: Oxford University Press. Pp. 135–150.

75. Stockley, A. V. (1969). "Computer Application in Radiation Dosimetry." In J. Rose (ed.), *Proceedings of the Symposium on Computers in Medicine.* London: J. & A. Churchill. Pp. 71–85.

76. Sletten, I. W., H. Altman, R. C. Evenson, and D. W. Cho (1973). "Computer Assignment of Psychotropic Drugs." *American Journal of Psychiatry,* **130**:595–598.

77. Bolinger, R. E., S. Price, and J. L. Kyner (1971). "Computerized Management of the Outpatient Diabetic." *Journal of the American Medical Association,* **216**:1779–1782.

78. *Medical World News* (1973). "Computerizing Drugs' Effect on Tests," **14**(18):71.

79. Wade, O. L. (1968). "The Computer and Drug Prescribing." In G. McLachlan, and R. A. Shegog (eds.), *Computers in the Service of Medicine: Essays on Current Research and Applications, Volume I.* London: Oxford University Press. Pp. 151–162.

80. Freud, S. (1950). *The Question of Lay Analysis: An Introduction to Psychoanalysis.* New York: Norton.

81. Malan, D. H. (1973). "The Outcome Problem in Psychotherapy Research: A Historical Review." *Archives of General Psychiatry,* **29**:719–729.

82. Ellul, J. (1964). *The Technological Society.* New York: Vintage.

83. Roszak, T. (1968). *The Making of the Counter Culture: Reflections on the Technocratic Society and Its Youthful Opposition.* Garden City, N. J.: Doubleday.

84. Sadler, A. M., Jr., B. L. Sadler, and A. A. Bliss (1972). *The Physician's Assistant: Today and Tomorrow.* New Haven: Yale University Press.

85. *Time* (1972). "The Return of the Midwife," **100**(21):56–58.

86. Lewis, F. J., S. Deller, M. Quinn, B. Lee, R. Will, and J. Raines (1972). "Continuous Patient Monitoring with A Small Digital Computer." *Computers and Biomedical Research,* **5**:411–428.

87. Bunker, J. P. (1970). "Surgical Manpower: A Comparison of Operations and Surgeons in the United States and in England and Wales." *New England Journal of Medicine,* **282**:135–144.

88. Greenberg, S. (1971). *The Quality of Mercy: A Report on the Critical Condition of Hospital and Medical Care in America.* New York: Atheneum.

89. Sedgwick, P. (1974). "Medical Individualism." *The Hastings Center Studies,* **2**(3):69–80.

90. Mechanic, D. (1972). *Public Expectations and Health Care: Essays on the Changing Organization of Health Services.* New York: Wiley-Interscience.

91. Bolande, R. P. (1969). "Ritualistic Surgery—Circumcision and Tonsilectomy." *New England Journal of Medicine,* **280**:591–596.

92. McCann, J. (1973). "Bile Acid Ingestion May Replace Some Surgery." *Biomedical News*, 4(10):6.

93. Field, M. G. (1971). "The Health Care System of Industrial Society: The Disappearance of the General Practitioner and Some Implications." In E. Mendelsohn, J. P. Swazey, and I. Taviss (eds.), *Human Aspects of Biomedical Innovation*. Cambridge: Harvard University Press. Pp. 156–180.

94. Tosteson, D. C. (1975). "What They're Saying. . ." *AAMC Educational News*, 2(3):6.

95. Korsch, B. M., and V. F. Neguete (1972). "Doctor-Patient Communication." *Scientific American*, 227(2):66–74.

96. Crowley, L. G., B. W. Nelson, and L. Aronow (1972). "How Stanford Selects New Medical Students." *Stanford M.D.*, 11(4):15–19.

97. Bradford, W. D. (1973). "Requirements for Admission to Medical School." In J. Graves (ed.), *The Future of Medical Education*. Durham, N. C.: Duke University Press. Pp. 53–69.

98. Mechanic, D. (1968). *Medical Sociology: A Selective View*. New York: Free Press.

99. Weed, L. L. (1969). *Medical Records, Medical Education, and Patient Care*. Cleveland: Press of Case Western Reserve University.

100. Stead, E. A., Jr. (1973). "Family Practice: One View." In J. Graves (ed.), *The Future of Medical Education*. Durham, N. C.: Duke University Press. Pp. 143–154.

101. Ehrlich, G. E. (1973). "Health Challenges of the Future." *The Annals of the American Academy of Political and Social Science*, 408:70–82.

102. Strauss, M. B. (ed.) (1968). *Familiar Medical Quotations*. Boston: Little, Brown.

103. Chase, A. (1971). *The Biological Imperatives: Health, Politics, and Human Survival*. Baltimore: Penguin.

104. Dubos, R. (1965). *Man Adapting*. New Haven: Yale University Press.

105. Thorner, R. M. (1969). "Whither Multiphasic Screening?" *New England Journal of Medicine*, 280:1037–1042.

106. Collen, M. F., P. H. Kidd, R. Feldman, and J. L. Cutler (1969). "Cost Analysis of A Multiphasic Screening Program." *New England Journal of Medicine*, 280:1043–1045.

107. *Kaiser Aluminum News* (1966). "She Had So Many Children. . ." 24(1): 10–13.

108. Ribicoff, A., and P. Danaceau (1973). *The American Medical Machine*. New York: Harrow.

109. London, I. M. (1973). "The College and University in Medical Education." In J. Graves (ed.), *The Future of Medical Education*. Durham, N. C.: Duke University Press. Pp. 43–51.

110. Van Der Kloot, W. G. (1973). "The Education of Biomedical Scientists." In J. Graves (ed.), *The Future of Medical Education*. Durham, N. C.: Duke University Press. Pp. 87–105.

111. Kiely, J. M., J. L. Juergens, B. L. Hisey, and P. E. Williams (1968). "A Computer-Based Medical Record: Entry of Data from the History and Physical Examination by the Physician." *Journal of the American Medical Association*, 205:571–576.

112. Dessau, E. (1969). "Hospital Information Systems-I." In J. F. Dickson, III, and J. H. U. Brown (eds.), *Future Goals of Engineering in Biology and Medicine*. New York: Academic. Pp. 251–267.

113. *Computers and Medicine* (1973). "MIS-1 After A Full Year's Operation— Pros & Cons," 2(6):1, 2, 4.

114. *Medical World News* (1972). "A Computerized Monitor to Screen Health Claims," 13(47):51.

115. Barnett, G. O. (1968). "Computers in Patient Care." *New England Journal of Medicine*, 279:1321–1327.

116. Levin, G., G. Hirsch, and E. Roberts (1971). "Narcotics and the Community: A Systems Simulation." *American Journal of Public Health*, 62: 861–873.

2

THE MYTH OF
PHYSICIAN NECESSITY _____

Man's strongest instinct is the will to live. We not only strive for longevity, but also crave a life free of infirmities. In the absence of health all human endeavors are compromised. Because health is a prerequisite for optimal achievement, the physician largely derives his preeminent status by virtue of his role as the protector of that health. Almost all of our aspirations and activities seem dependent upon the continued existence of the doctor. To propose and advocate that we deliberately plan for the obsolescence of the physician may appear to be tantamount to abnegating the significance of our very health and survival. The myth of physician necessity reigns unchallenged within a society that is preoccupied with its physical and psychological well-being. I maintain, however, that in the future our health will not be contingent upon the continued presence of the doctor. The emergence of a Post-Physician Era will enhance the vitality of our citizenry and thereby enrich the quality of human existence.

In suggesting that doctors can and should be replaced by a medic-computer symbiosis, I do not wish to minimize the vital skills and accomplishments of contemporary physicians. Without their clinical efforts and scientific discoveries, without their willingness to use allied health professionals and computers in clinical practice, a Post-Physician Era could never become a viable alternative future. Although physicians may unwittingly hasten their own obsolescence, this fact should in no way denigrate their significant role in medical history. If a medic-computer model of health care delivery is to be a possible, inevitable, and desirable alternative medical future, doctors who have contributed to its development will deserve our gratitude. Nevertheless, the myth of physician necessity must be refuted.

INTUITION VERSUS LOGIC.   Many individuals believe that the computer will be unable to replicate the intellectual capacities of the doctor. Although generally it is acknowledged that the decision making processes of the physician are poorly understood (1), the assumption that he blends a combination of *intuition* and *logic* in reaching diagnostic and treatment conclusions is reasonable. So intermeshed are these two qualities that doctors themselves are unable to determine which of them predominates in performing their clinical activities. Webster defines intuition as "the power or faculty of attaining to direct knowledge or cognition without rational thought and inference." Based upon his experiences of himself and the world he inhabits, man's use of intuition involves the use of his feelings and sensitivities. We exalt this power of intuition. In an age increasingly dominated by the machine, our intuition seems to distinguish us from the machine. Many authors have stated that the physician's intuitive abilities not only differentiate him from the computer, but also provide him with an unassailable advantage over it (2–3). So pervasive is this assumption that it is rarely, if ever, seriously challenged.

In former times priests, barber-surgeons, apothecaries, and lay practitioners favorably competed with doctors as the providers of health care. All of these healers sought to cure the afflicted with their intuitive sense of what they felt would restore the physical

well-being of their clientele. Despite their sincere and often
zealous efforts, their results were at best erratic. The physician's
use of logic, rather than of intuition, elevated him to his position
as the exclusive authority on medical matters. Eliot Freidson has
shown that the ascendance of the medical profession evolved only
after physicians adopted the scientific method as a way of
contending with clinical problems (4). The populace realized
that, unlike the methods utilized by other practitioners, the
techniques performed by the scientifically oriented physician
worked. When faced with the appalling rate of infant mortality
in colonial Massachusetts, even the reverend Cotton Mather, who
counseled submission to God's will as the true path to the salvation of the body, resorted to the prescriptions of scientific medicine
(5).

That physicians utilize intuition is indisputable; that this
intuition usually helps the patient, however, is doubtful. We
often make the mistaken assumption that the doctor's intuition is
correct. In truth the physician's intuition is always affected by his
feelings toward the patient, his temperament, and the tensions he
experiences as a result of the taxing nature of his work. All of
these factors distort his clinical objectivity. A doctor's intuition
can be wrong as often as it is right. This fact is not reassuring; it
is not meant to be. Applied by an artist, subjectivity can lead to an
aesthetic masterpiece; applied by a physician, it can lead to
further illness or even death. In attempting to justify the superiority of the doctor's intuition over the computer's logic, David
Rutstein offers us the following example: "Indeed the 'sick
headache' of a nervous, middle-aged woman without serious
illness may be described in more vivid terms than may the
headache due to a brain tumor in a stoic patient. History taking. . .
is far removed from being amenable to programming on a
computer" (6, p. 104). This view exemplifies the very dangerous,
albeit pervasive, faith in the doctor's intuitive capacity to distinguish between "real" and "imaginary" disease. Too many
patients with serious medical illnesses are misdiagnosed as having
simple anxiety (7). Although Rutstein's nervous middle-aged
woman may in fact be nervous, she may also have a brain tumor.

Only the use of rigorous medical logic can lead us to the correct diagnosis.

Of course the doctor's intuitively derived conclusions prove to be justified at times. But even in these circumstances his decisions are not based upon random guesswork; instead they represent a less than fully conscious awareness of the logical steps needed to reach the correct determination. Once the logical pathways in this seemingly intuitive process can be understood and specified, they can be and have been programmed into a computer (8–10). Physicians' use of intuition is no justification for their continued existence; for it is their logical rather than their intuitive thought processes that lead to accurate clinical decision making.

THE DOCTOR AND THE COMPUTER: A TECHNICAL COMPARISON. Although the doctor's use of logic enables him to reach accurate clinical determinations and the computer cannot be anything but logical, we should not assume automatically that computers possess the capacity or the versatility required to exceed the physician's ability to render logical medical decisions. In fact, many developers of computerized methods routinely add the proviso that their systems are intended to assist rather than to replace the physician (1, 11–12). In doing so they raise a multiplicity of *allegedly* technical limitations to the clinical use of medical computers and thereby imply that the continued existence of the physician is inevitable. A closer examination of the subject, however, may lead us to the opposite conclusion.

Three major capabilities are required for logical medical decisions—*objectivity*, *probability*, and *memory*. By recognizing that the machine can outperform the doctor in conducting each of these tasks, the advantages of the computer begin to become apparent. The statement that the physician's subjectivity often leads to inaccurate clinical determinations is not meant to be a condemnation of doctors. It only is intended to show that, as human beings, physicians can be unduly influenced by their feelings and can make serious errors in judgment (13). Regardless of how much the doctor strives to be objective, he can never equal the rationality of the computer (14). Every clinical decision rendered by the physician also necessitates a consideration of probabilities. For example, a coughing patient has a greater chance of having a cold than of having lung cancer. Over the years the doctor acquires a sense of which symptoms and signs in a particular group of individuals are most likely to be manifestations of a certain disease. In reaching these decisions the physician's knowledge is limited to what he has learned from his training, reading, and experience. The totality of this information, although impressive, can never equal the collective wisdom of all physicians. The typical doctor may be proficient at recognizing and treating routine ailments, but he is less acquainted with rare disorders (12). No doctor can know everything (15). But the computer of the future will have an almost unlimited storage capacity (16), and, therefore, could amass all available medical knowledge. It could be programmed to render decisions about *all* diseases, whether common or exotic (17). Because the machine could possess a considerably larger amount of information than could the physician, it would have a greater ability to determine accurate diagnostic and treatment probabilities. Similarly, whereas the doctor's capacity to remember and draw upon relevant medical data is limited, the computer's ability to memorize and release information would be almost infinite (13). Whether we like it or not, the machine's capacity to remember cannot be doubted. As Matthew Dumont has said, 'Computers are machines which cannot forget. Therein lies the new divinity. The Gods of Olympus could forget, so could the God of Abraham, Isaac, and Jacob. And Jesus and Buddha and the others. They were all capable of forgetting. Not our machines; *they never forget*" (Dumont's italics) (18, p. 7). The computer readily surpasses the physician in objectivity, probability, and memory. *

The question if computers can replicate the exact means by which doctors make decisions is irrelevant. That the thought

---

* More technical discussions of the theoretical issues involved in the medical application of computers can be found elsewhere (1–2, 19–20).

processes of the physician are mediated by biochemical interactions and the calculations of the computer are performed by
electronic mechanisms does not tell us anything about their
comparative abilities to render accurate clinical determinations.
Instead, the critical issue is if the computer and the doctor can
reach identical conclusions, regardless of how they get there
(1, 21–22)* When studies have been conducted comparing the
diagnostic accuracy of the machine to that of the physician, the
former generally have approximated and at times even exceeded
the ability of the latter (13, 17, 23–28).† The belief that computers do not "think" is besides the point in assessing the utility
of automated medical decision making.

Of course the machine's ability to offer reliable judgments is
only as good as the program it utilizes. As computer technologists
are fond of saying, "garbage in—garbage out." If a medical
computer is fed a poorly designed or invalid program, its decisions
will reflect these errors. Conversely, if a machine possesses an
accurate program, it can generate worthwhile conclusions. When
the logical pathways needed to make a diagnosis are delineated,
they readily can be and have been programmed into the computer.
Unfortunately, at present the logical pathways required to diagnose many ailments have not been identified. Until this occurs the
computer will be unable to make reliable decisions. To expect
that in the future medical scientists will be able to formulate
these logical pathways is reasonable. But even if these pathways
cannot be delineated for certain diseases, the computer will

* No two physicians utilize identical thought processes in making clinical
decisions, even though they often will reach the same conclusion.
† The issue of comparing the doctor's diagnostic ability to that of the computer
is more complex than one might imagine. Very often the physicians who program the computer are the same ones who serve as the comparison group.
Therefore, it is not surprising that in these circumstances the agreement rate
between man and machine is very high. Furthermore, who is correct when a
doctor and a computer disagree over the interpretation of, for example, an
EKG? Because findings from other more sophisticated cardiac studies, open
heart surgery, and even an autopsy may be inconclusive, the issue of whether
the computer or the physician was correct frequently remains unresolved (29).
Nevertheless, there are strong indications that the machine can diagnose as well
as if not better than the doctor.

be in no worse position than the physician in providing accurate determinations (13). For example, in one study of psychiatric patients the rate of diagnostic agreement between the computer and the clinician was only 50 to 60 percent. However, in the same study the authors noted that the rate of agreement between psychiatrists was also only 50 to 60 percent (23). This investigation neither invalidates the clinical utility of computers nor casts aspersions on the clinicians who diagnosed these patients, for the determination of psychiatric diagnoses is notoriously unreliable (30). This lack of agreement is hardly limited to psychiatrists; it prevails among all medical specialists (31). Whether utilized by a machine or by a physician, inadequate or poorly understood diagnostic criteria often lead to unreliable conclusions. Computerized medical decision making is limited in the same areas in which the doctor is also unable to reach accurate diagnostic and treatment determinations (13, 28).

Other critics have suggested that unlike a physician, a computer would be unable to diagnose a patient from "scratch." When a patient initially sees a doctor, the physician must determine from among numerous possibilities the specific disease or diseases that are afflicting his client. Generally, the doctor is able to narrow quickly the range of possibilities by making "intuitive leaps"—a process the computer is unable to perform. It has been argued that because the machine could not possess an adequate storage capacity or be sufficiently selective in making its observations, it would be unable to diagnose a newly presenting patient (2). However, because computer storage capacity has been expanding by a factor of 10 every two to three years (32), medical computers will not be limited by this consideration. Although machines cann t distinguish between relevant and extraneous data, evidence suggests that diagnoses can be made from "scratch." A study was conducted in which the Cornell Medical Index, a 195-item questionnaire, was administered to 5929 consecutively hospitalized patients. A machine analyzed the questionnaires to yield a diagnosis from among 60 possibilities. The result of this investigation revealed that the machine-derived diagnoses were slightly more accurate than those rendered by physicians (25).

Any system of health care delivery that would rely heavily upon the computer would have to include consideration of a number of geographic and temporal parameters. Because certain diseases are more common in some areas than in others, computer probabilities would have to be adjusted to reflect the prevalence of a disorder in a particular region (1, 20). A single computer program could not be applied universally; it would have to be modified selectively to conform to local conditions (33). Furthermore, the rate of occurrence of certain illnesses changes. For example, the incidence of syphilis has fluctuated markedly throughout the 20th century (34), and other illnesses, such as the flu, vary on a seasonal basis. An effective diagnostic computer would have to be adjusted to reflect these variations (19–20). Whereas computer programs can be updated easily and rapidly to respond to changing conditions, often physicians are unfamiliar with these important geographical and temporal factors.

These variables are not the only ones that affect automated diagnosis. A more complicated problem emerges when a patient has not one but rather two or more coexisting illnesses. Some authors have suggested that the computer would be unable to discern if the patient's symptoms are the manifestations of a single or numerous diseases (2). However, the problem of multiple diagnoses represents an equally complex dilemma for both the physician and the computer (1). Nevertheless, if the logical pathways by which a doctor diagnoses simultaneously occurring illnesses can be delineated, this problem should not represent an obstacle to providing reliable automated decision making. In fact, computers already have been programmed to diagnose two or more concurrently existing disorders (35–36).

Closely related to the question of multiple diagnoses is the issue of "relative risk." For example, a computer may determine that a patient has a 70 percent chance of having disease A and a 20 percent chance of having disease B. In most circumstances one would first treat disease A and only treat disease B if disease A did not respond to the proper therapy. Although disease A is the most likely disorder affecting the patient, disease B could be considerably more dangerous. In this case should one initially treat the relatively benign, but more likely, disease A or the more serious, but less probable, disease B? Some authors have suggested that computer determined treatments would be unable to resolve this dilemma (2). The issue of "relative risk" presents an equally vexing problem for both the doctor and the computer. The physician is faced with this dilemma every day, and despite whatever uncertainty he may experience, he forges ahead and selects a particular treatment. Regardless of which disease he chooses to treat, his ultimate judgment is rendered after weighing the relative merits of embarking upon either course of action. His decision is based upon probabilities, a function that is well-suited to the computer. The problem of "relative risk" could be resolved more productively by a machine than by a physician.

The computer could overcome another grave problem in our present physician-centered model of health care delivery. Although there are more than one billion patient–doctor contacts per year in the United States alone (37), only a minute amount of data obtained from these visits is ever used to benefit medical science. The overwhelming majority of clinical observations remain with the practicing physician and are never conveyed to researchers who could utilize this information to acquire a fuller understanding of disease. One of the greatest obstacles to providing optimal patient care is that we do not possess an adequate data base upon which to make useful diagnostic and treatment decisions. If all clinical observations were automated, the computer could generate this data so that researchers could advance our medical knowledge (13) and significantly improve patient care.

Even among those individuals who recognize the numerous advantages of medical computers, many assert that "the best" physician will always surpass the performance of "the best" computer. This belief would be true if the doctor's tasks were restricted to supportive and psychotherapeutic functions. In the future, however, these responsibilities could be assumed by a medic, who in contrast to the contemporary doctor, would be able to focus primarily upon these activities. In terms of the more technical functions of the physician, the best computer could at least equal the performance of the best doctor. The best physician could delineate his logical decision making processes and have them programmed into a computer (10). Even if one accepts the dubious assumption that the best doctor can surpass the best computer, the fact is that truly great physicians are exceedingly rare. Doctors range from the brilliant to the dangerous. In contrast to these varying levels of competence, properly programmed computers could provide the highest available quality of clinical decision making. Unlike our present physician-centered system, a medic-computer model could provide *all* patients with the most expert medical care.

Even the best doctors make mistakes. Physicians are human. They become tired, bored, grouchy, and forgetful (13). The persistent tensions and excessive demands that accompany the practice of medicine cannot help but adversely affect the quality of their work. Properly programmed computers do not make mistakes. Although we are delighted whenever we hear of a computer making a spectacular blunder, in truth the fault lies not with the machine but with the man who programmed it.

One could state that physicians have an advantage over machines in the sense that doctors can learn from experience and computers cannot. Physicians theoretically can increase their clinical skills every day they practice, and updating a computer on a daily basis may be difficult. This alleged advantage of the physician is based on the assumption that, unlike the doctor, the computer cannot learn from experience. The literature on artificial intelligence, however, would suggest the opposite (21).

The most illustrious example of a computer that learns from experience is Arthur Samuel's checker playing machine. Although initially his computer was hardly able to beat a child, the machine was programmed to store the sequences of plays that resulted in capturing its opponent's pieces. With each subsequent game the computer compared the existing pattern of play with the many patterns it had memorized. It then chose a move that its experience had demonstrated would most likely lead to victory. Eventually the machine not only was able to beat Samuel, who considers himself a "fair amateur," but other experts as well (21, 38–40).

Theoretically, if a computer can learn from its checker playing experience, it also should be able to learn from its experience in treating patients. Every time a computer generates a treatment decision, the results of that decision could be fed back into the machine. Eventually the computer could learn from its "clinical experience" and automatically update its own program. A "self-educating" medical computer has not yet been developed, but one can anticipate that by the year 2000 computers that learn from experience will be widely available (32). A medical computer that learns while it treats would be a vast improvement over many physicians, who over the years develop a kind of intellectual anesthesia. Instead of continually learning from their patient care experiences, they seem to stagnate and rely upon outmoded clinical methods. Only some physicians continue to learn; in the future all medical computers could possess this trait.

Of course there is a considerable difference between something being theoretically feasible and commercially available. Today computer technology has not been developed sufficiently to provide clinical services on an extensive basis. A lack of storage capacity, effective diagnostic and treatment programs, precise medical terminology, and accessible hardware are only a few of the obstacles that must be overcome before computers can be used widely in the delivery of health care services. But that is not to say that these technical problems cannot be overcome. Since the introduction of the first electronic digital computer in 1944 (41), the efficiency, capacity, and versatility of the machine has evolved to such an extent that even some of the most optimistic observers have underestimated its rate of development (16). There is every reason to believe that this progress will continue as we move toward the 21st century. Therefore, if a medic-computer model of health care delivery fails to come about, it will not be because we lack the technical abilities to accomplish this objective.

SOCIOECONOMIC CONTINGENCIES. To a large extent the emergence of a Post-Physician Era will be contingent upon the existence of a favorable economic and social climate. Technological innovations will be developed and applied extensively only within a society that commits its fiscal human, and institutional resources to attaining these goals (42–43).

The financial expenditures that would be required to create a medic-computer model would be enormous. The initial cost of developing computer programs and facilities has been one of the major obstacles to the widespread application of automated techniques in clinical medicine (9, 44). Nevertheless, economic considerations will not necessarily prevent the attainment of a Post-Physician Era. Although present costs vary considerably, in one computerized history system that takes 82 minutes to complete, the price averaged $4.25 per interview during weekdays and half that amount during evenings and weekends (13). (Compared to physician's fees, this is a real bargain.) Furthermore, most experts anticipate that the costs of computer equipment will continue to decline. Within the past 15 years the expense of automated computations has decreased by a factor of 1000 (45). In the future, for the equivalent of only a few dollars a month, individuals will have a vast array of computer services at their disposal (16, 46). The establishment of economical computer utilities could provide medical, as well as educational and commercial benefits. These lowered costs will be possible in part because computers will become mass produced, utilize "time-sharing," and possess greater storage and retrieval capacities (16).

From a strictly financial perspective, we may be unable *not* to afford an automated medical care system. Although developing computerized methods are highly expensive, so too is the present system by which we educate physicians. For example, in 1972 it cost between $50,600 and $104,000 to train only *one* medical student (47). These figures do *not* include the funds needed to support the physician's pre- and postmedical school education. Furthermore, primarily because of inflation, tuitions have more than doubled in the past decade (48). At the same time, because medical knowledge has been rapidly increasing, the period required of doctors to complete their postgraduate specialty training has also been expanding. Thus, by the time a doctor actually completes his formal training, he is able to practice for only approximately 35 years. Surveys indicate that although doctors currently spend 46.9 hours per week in direct patient contact (37), 67 percent of physicians believe that by 1978 this time will decrease by as much as 33 percent (49). As a result, doctors will be treating a fewer number of individuals. Therefore, when comparing the limited time physicians will be delivering clinical services to the exorbitant costs of training them to do so, a physician-centered model is hardly an economical one.

Under our present system of medical care, the available supply of doctors within a society needs constant replenishment, and therefore, financing the training of new physicians is perpetual. Once a medical computer program has been devised, it can be transferred to and utilized by other computers throughout the country. This can be accomplished with minimal difficulty and at a nominal expense (33). Consequently, high quality technical medical decision making can be made available to a much greater number of patients than can be serviced by a multitude of physicians. Despite the initial high cost of developing an automated health care system, in the long run it may prove to be a financially advantageous approach.

But even if it is not, providing medical services cannot be determined *solely* by those with an "econo-think" mentality. While we strive to economize on the delivery of clinical services, we must not abandon or forget other human values, such as the need to enhance the health of the populace. Although we cannot ignore fiscal considerations, neither can we afford to be guided exclusively by them.

Whether sufficient funds will be allocated to support the development of a medic-computer model will depend largely upon future government economic policies. Unfortunately, the vicissitudes of politics do not allow a forecaster to render accurate predictions about anticipated fiscal priorities. For instance, since the end of World War II, federal funds for medical research catapulted nearly 200 times. However, with the advent of a series of events that were unrelated to the public's desire for improved health care (e.g., the Vietnam War, the election of Richard

Nixon), this trend was suddenly reversed (50). This example illustrates two points: First, it is difficult to make long-range plans when a government's fiscal priorities are perpetually changing. Second, politicians, who are charged with the task of allocating money for health care, often are elected on the basis of issues that are totally unrelated to medicine. As a result, it is nearly impossible to offer accurate long-range forecasts of government expenditures for medical research, education, and service.

Mark Field has noted that regardless of the vital significance of medical care, ". . .the health system does *not* stand at the center of the societal universe around which everything else should revolve" (Field's italics) (51). Medicine will continually have to compete with national defense, housing, welfare, foreign aid, and so on for scarce federal dollars. Furthermore, even within medicine fierce competition for government funds exists. Should automated health care systems receive priority over other important demands, such as expanding medical education, pre-natal care, basic science, or clinical research (52–53)? These are difficult issues to work out, but their ultimate resolution may determine when and if a medic-computer model will be actualized.

The decisions about government health expenditures will be affected by the lobbying efforts of organized medicine. There are strong indications that if present trends continue, physicians will have less authority over the allocation of federal funds for health care delivery and medical research (43). The doctor–patient relationship is being superseded by a tripartite relationship in which the state assumes ultimate responsibility for patient care (54). Furthermore, not only has the American Medical Association's (AMA) virtual monopoly over health legislation declined, but so too has its control over the medical profession it purports to represent. In 1959 fifty-nine percent of American doctors were dues-paying members of the AMA (55); by 1975 this figure had dropped to 41 percent (56). Whether this trend will persist or reverse remains to be seen. But regardless of the size of its membership, those who belong to the AMA increasingly do not subscribe to the organization's conservative political philosophy. Although exact statistics are unavailable, many doctors are almost and at times actually forced to join the AMA or its constituent societies to acquire hospital privileges, state licensure, or malpractice insurance (57).

The relative declining number of doctors within the health care industry and among the intellectual elite has also served to reduce the power of physicians over the politics of health care delivery. In 1900 sixty-seven percent of medical personnel were physicians. Today less than 10 percent of medical personnel are physicians. Furthermore, the ratio of doctors to other members of the educational elite has decreased. In 1900 there were five physicians to every one college faculty member. In 1970 there was one physician to every two college faculty members (58). If all of these trends persist, doctors will have a progressively decreasing influence over government medical programs and will be in less of a position to prevent their own obsolescence.

Legal precedents also may promote the implementation of a medic-computer model. Physicians, concerned about malpractice, are aware that they can be sued if they do not practice medicine according to the *normative standards* of care provided by doctors in the same field within their community (59). Unlike several decades ago, today the failure to order certain ancillary tests could render the physician susceptible to a malpractice suit. As computerized medical decision making becomes more widely available, a physician who fails to consult an automated system also may be legally liable. Forensic considerations may "encourage" doctors to accept the use of computers and, therefore, accelerate the emergence of a Post-Physician Era.

Medicine's future will be guided by a complex interplay of rational, semirational, and nonrational forces. The technical considerations previously mentioned constitute the rational elements of the equation; the socioeconomic factors briefly described in this section represent the semirational parts of the formula. I have restricted my discussion of these later variables to the extent that they support the contention that a medic-computer model is possible, desirable, and inevitable. Other significant social, political, and economic parameters that will affect the future of medicine are examined in the following chapter. Before exploring them, however, we need to look at the nonrational elements of the equation; for the inner needs, fears, and hopes of man will help to shape the future as much as, if not more than, the technological, social, political, and economic forces that exist outside of him.

PSYCHOHISTORICAL CONSIDERATIONS. Historically, massive public outcries have accompanied technological innovations. In 19th-century England bands of workers known as Luddites destroyed the newly introduced textile machines. Today, the adversaries of technology are equally visible and vocal (60–62). These Neo-Luddites raise a number of legitimate, and not so legitimate, doubts about our increasingly automated society. Regardless of the merits of their arguments, their concerns are pervasive because they resound with some of the deepest fears of contemporary man.

Although a comprehensive summary of the psychological attitudes toward technology is beyond the scope of this book,* several factors are mentioned frequently. People do not understand computers; they feel estranged from and controlled by those who do. Others are terrified by the rapid changes brought on by the introduction of automated systems and fear that their livelihoods will be endangered. The spectres of living in and being totally dependent upon an artificial environment haunt those who seek to escape from what they feel is rapidly becoming a dehumanized society. While some decry the power of technology, others are resentful because it is not powerful enough. We expect our machines to solve all of our wartime problems— whether it be a military war or a war on poverty, overpopulation, or disease. In former times an almighty God was the recipient of man's personal frustrations; today the almighty Computer has become his scapegoat. Contemporary man is ambivalent about his technology; he dreads its mythical omnipotence yet resents its inevitable deficiencies.

---

* More extensive discussions of this topic can be found elsewhere (16, 18, 62–64).

The atmosphere of suspicion that envelops our attitudes about technology undoubtedly will influence our society's readiness to replace the "black bag" with the "black box." Our reluctance to accept the myth of physician necessity lies not only in our distrust of technology, but also in our eternal wish to deify the physician. Of all the ancient arts, only medicine produced a god—Aesculapius. Despite the increasing secularization of society, we continue to exalt our physicians, although we do so in a peculiar fashion. We hear a great deal about impersonal, profit-seeking doctors, but they usually seem to be somebody else's doctor, not our own. We tend to criticize physicians, not as we know them, but rather by what we know *about* them. When our very personal health and survival depend upon a doctor, that doctor assumes godlike dimensions. Modern man, however, is fickle in his choice of deities. A mere 50 years ago the proclamation that God is dead was viewed as the invective of an apostate. Today this notion is fashionable even among theologians. The public's recognition of the exceptional abilities of the computer to deliver medical care may result in our declining need to exalt the physician. If this occurs, *the machine may replace the doctor as the primary object of man's apparent need to deify a healer*. To justify this assertion, one needs to examine the psychological forces that have shaped our attitudes toward those individuals who throughout history have functioned as healers. The following explanations are based largely upon psychoanalytic theory and, therefore, must be considered as speculations rather than as facts.

Because the doctor is the guardian of man's intense desire to live, he is seen as having a vital role within our society. This reasoning, however, is not fully satisfactory. It explains why the doctor is needed, but not why he is exalted. It explains our need to view him as important, but not our need to view him as omnipotent. One may obtain insight into the question of why man tends to ascribe godlike qualities to the physician by considering certain preconscious and unconscious psychodynamic forces. *

* In Freudian terminology *preconscious material* refers to all mental activity that

Patients *wish* the doctor to possess three interrelated traits: 1. *Reliability*. They want to feel that the physician will always be available especially during moments of distress. They also hope that he will relate to them in a reasonably consistent manner. Erratic, unpredictable behavior from a physician raises the spectre of the unknown, which in turn increases the anxiety they already experience from knowing they are sick. 2. *Nurturance*. Patients want the doctor to act with sympathy, compassion, and even tenderness. Although most patients would never say so, they yearn for the physician to cater to and satisfy their every desire. One of the social consequences of illness is that patients expect the doctor to ensure that all of their physical and emotional needs (i.e., food, clothes, shelter, psychological support) will be provided for by someone other than the patient (4, 31). 3. *Omnipotence*. Patients want to have complete faith that their physician knows all and, more important, can accomplish all. They wish to be absolutely confident that under no circumstances could their doctor ever make a mistake. Although no one seriously expects the physician to possess all of these virtues, this realistic assessment in no way deters patients from *wishing* that their doctor has these qualities. To varying degrees, patients are in a state of *dependency* and want *protection* from all internal and external stresses.

That these psychological characteristics of patients approximate closely the characteristics of infancy and early childhood might be more than coincidental. The infant, who exists in a state of total or near total dependency, seeks protection from all forms of discomfort (65). He wants his mother or mother-surrogate to be reliable; she must be everpresent and always consistent. Erik Erikson has emphasized this quality by suggesting that it is during infancy that we acquire or fail to acquire a sense of *basic trust* in others (66). Throughout infancy the child is dependent upon the nurturance of others. He needs to be clothed, fed, and hugged. Once the infant is able to distinguish between self and

---

is "out of mind" but can be recalled with minimal effort or stimulation. *Unconscious material* refers to all mental activity that not only is "out of mind" but also can be revealed to consciousness only under certain types of severe emotional strain or via psychoanalysis.

nonself, he gradually begins to believe in parental omnipotence. Although this belief develops more fully in later life, the child recognizes that mother can give or remove food, alleviate or cause pain, provide or deny warmth (65). Finally, to survive, the relatively helpless infant requires and demands protection by those in his environment.

Because they are acquired during the initial stage of life, infantile experiences serve as the lattice work upon which all subsequent experiences are built. In later life, as our dependency lessens and our need for protection by others diminishes, the necessity to have reliable, nurturant, and omnipotent figures is also decreased. However, when one is ill, strong dependency needs similar to those experienced in infancy become resurrected, and the patient seeks protection by his physician in a manner resembling his childhood desire for maternal protection. The patient's quest for a reliable, nurturant, and omnipotent doctor derives not only from his present, legitimate, and conscious needs, but also from a recrudescence of his powerful unconscious infantile wishes. Moreover, his need to exalt rather than simply to admire the physician may partially stem from these earlier life experiences. Although other factors, such as cultural norms, reality circumstances, and previous encounters with doctors, shape his attitudes toward the physician, the interpretation of these variables is also greatly influenced by his infantile experiences.

The person expected to gratify a patient's quest for an omnipotent, nurturant, and reliable healer has changed throughout history according to the prevailing ideologies of the day. Based upon theological beliefs, ancient man looked to the shaman or the priest to alleviate his infirmities. Today man's faith in science allows him to trust the ministrations of the physician. Tomorrow man's awesome respect for technology may encourage him to depend upon the computer to fulfill his medical needs.

We are entering a psychohistorical era in which we are ascribing to and expecting the computer to gratify our dependency strivings. The fact that modern man expresses an intense dislike for and suspicion of technology does not negate this hypothesis. Whether it is God, shaman, or physician, throughout history man always has had strong ambivalent feelings toward the objects of their infantile-derived quest for omnipotent, nurturant, and reliable figures.

How, then, can one tell which is the dominant side of man's ambivalence? One looks at what man does, not at what he says, and what he does is to allow technology to encroach upon every sphere of human activity. Contrary to the paranoid fantasies of some, the growth of automation is not the plot of a technocratic elite. The psychological impetus behind the expansion of technology lies in contemporary man's belief in the machine's capacities for omnipotence, nurturance, and reliability. Man cannot avoid ascribing omnipotence to the computer. Every day he reads about machines assuming tasks that once only man himself could perform. The image of the omnipotent computer is reinforced by the aura of complexity, and thereby mystery, that enshrouds the machine. Although a programmer can err, the computer cannot. Consequently, the belief in the reliability of the machine reigns unchallenged. True, the computer cannot provide warmth and tenderness, * but it is becoming an indispensable tool in caring for human needs. It issues our pay checks, guides our policy makers, teaches our children, and regulates our activities (41, 67). I am not suggesting that the computer necessarily *is* omnipotent, reliable, or caring. What I am suggesting, however, is that from a psychological perspective we yearn for and believe that the machine can manifest these qualities. If this assumption is correct, shamans, physicians, and computers share certain fundamental characteristics—namely, they have been and are the recipients of man's infantile-derived needs for omnipotent, nurturant, and reliable figures. In the future patients will be psychologically prepared to transfer their godlike respect for the doctor to the machine.

Some readers may feel that this hypothesis is overly speculative. They may argue that common sense dictates that people will

---

* One even could take issue with this statement by predicting that in the future children will extensively utilize the computer for entertainment, education, and emotional feedback. Already television, another product of technology, has become America's number one mother-surrogate.

never accept the machine as a substitute for the physician, and therefore, a medic-computer model could never materialize. This conviction does not imply satisfaction with our present health care system—its deficiencies are well known—yet many individuals prefer to live with familiar problems—rather than to contend with new solutions. To avoid the emotional turmoil that accompanies rapid social change, they seek to resurrect the past (38). For example, the naive belief exists that the inadequacies of our health care system can be rectified by reviving the old-time general practitioner (58, 68–69). The many advocates of this superficially appealing idea can be found among health care planners, medical educators, and the general public. To illustrate how enraptured some individuals are with this proposal, the University of Michigan actually invited Robert Young who portrays Dr. Marcus Welby, to speak at their medical school commencement. (It is unfortunate, but revealing, that to display someone who exemplifies the ideal family physician, the school had to choose an actor instead of a doctor.)

In theory, the revitalized general practitioner would be trained to deal with common diseases as well as to recognize and refer patients with more unusual disorders. However, these tasks apparently are being performed with nearly equal skill by physician's assistants, nurse-clinicians, and nurse-practitioners (70–72). Why train a doctor to do what a paraprofessional can do at considerably less expense? Even if one still desires to retain the general practitioner, to expect that he can practice high quality medicine is unreasonable. Specialization did not evolve by accident; it occurred largely because there simply was too much knowledge for a general practitioner to assimilate if he was to provide clinical excellence. Although most authorities would acknowledge his relative lack of technical skill, they feel that at least the general practitioner could offer mediocre care with tenderness and compassion (68). I fail, however, to see the virtue of a healer who is unable to heal. If you die as a result of his incompetence, who cares that he holds your hand as you expire? Well-intended priests and bartenders could do as well.

Even if we could tolerate his technical ineptitude, we should not accept automatically the mythology that he was universally loved and idolized by his patients. We have forgotten that for centuries most physicians rarely, if ever, saw a patient. While they were preoccupied with science or theology, the healing arts were performed mainly by shamans, barbers, apothecaries, and lay-practitioners. There were, of course, exceptions, but the history of doctors is usually the history of *great* doctors, and only a few of them treated the sick (4). When they did, they were ridiculed and scorned as often as they were respected and adored. On his deathbed Alexander the Great said, "I die by the help of too many physicians" (73, p. 257). Molière viewed doctors as avaricious, bumbling buffoons. Thomas Jefferson was highly skeptical of the healing arts, including the practices of his friend Dr. Benjamin Rush. Jefferson once said that whenever he saw two doctors conversing, he scanned the sky for an approaching buzzard (74). William Douglass, an outstanding mid-18th century physician, depicted the doctor's clinical activities as "an impudent delusion and a fraud" (5, p. 469). A hundred years later a widely read and accepted study of the medical profession observed: "The science of patient-getting is often more assiduously studied than that of patient-curing. Real success is not so much desired as the mere appearance of it" (75, p. 16). At least until this century, physicians were often seen as hucksters instead of as healers. To romanticize the past is understandable, but to resurrect it would be un-pardonable.

We not only have glorified yesterday's doctor, we have over-estimated today's physician. Frequently we assume that the improved health of our populace has resulted primarily from his diligent efforts. There is ample evidence, however, that good nutrition, adequate housing, and effective sanitation have contributed more to the emergence of a healthy citizenry than all of the doctor's clinical activities (76). We also tend to ignore the degree to which the physician is dependent upon technology. Divest him of his sophisticated laboratory tests, X-rays, EKGs, and medications, and his clinical utility would be severely reduced. The effectiveness of the contemporary doctor lies primarily in his use of technology, rather than in his innate ability to heal. Failing to appreciate this distinction, modern man continues to deify the physician.

That patients will ever abandon the doctor and entrust their health to a medic-computer symbiosis may seem unlikely. One reason that people are reluctant to accept an automated system of health care delivery is because they are unaccustomed to computers; they seem too complex, awesome, and mysterious. Nevertheless, familiarity tends to breed acceptance. Increasingly, computers will become an integral part of our daily lives (16, 38, 46). As this occurs, the enigmatic image of the computer will subside, and gradually we will feel less estranged from using it. The acclimatization process has already begun. While many youngsters are using automated systems in their schools, others are playing with toy computers in their homes. Tomorrow's children will grow up with computers, just as today's children have grown up with television. Consequently, future generations will feel at ease with the machine and be more likely to trust it to make significant medical decisions.

As these systems become more widely available and patients recognize their clinical utility, they will expect to be interviewed by a computer in much the same way that they currently expect to receive a physical examination. Patient acceptance of auto-mated history takers has been high in clinical settings where it has been tried (11, 13, 77–83). Although results vary, patients generally have preferred computerized histories over those gathered by physicians. For example, Slack et al. found that 36 percent of patients with allergies favored a history taken by a machine, while 24 percent preferred one taken by a doctor. The remaining 40 percent had no preference. Nearly all of these patients found giving a history to the computer an interesting and enjoyable experience (80). At the Massachusetts General Hospital 35 percent favored automated histories, while 33 percent preferred to speak with a physician. The others did not express a preference. The question might arise if the relatively positive attitudes of patients toward computerized histories is a reflection of the novelty of the experience rather than a genuine desire to interact with the machine. In this latter study 54 percent of patients were found to be willing to talk to a medical computer in the future, while 23 percent would not. Twenty-three percent had no preference (79). These investigations seem to indicate that the frequently expressed argument that computerized history taking would be "dehumanizing" does not seem to bear up—at least according to the patients who actually have utilized the machine. One might claim that psychiatric patients would be more sensitive to and distressed by automated history gathering than would general medical patients. Studies do not confirm this belief. In one investigation 52 percent of suicidal patients preferred to offer their histories to a computer (13). Half of the mothers of emotionally disturbed children felt that communicating with a machine was as easy as speaking with their doctor; 37.5 percent thought it was harder; 67.5 percent claimed they were as frank with the computer as they usually were with their psychiatrist; and 15 percent felt they could be more honest with the machine (78). When asked to compare his experiences with both the computer and his doctor, one psychiatric patient said, 'It feels good to talk to something that doesn't talk back" (82). Although most patients have accepted the computer, others have not, but patients are hardly unanimous in accepting their doctors either (41, 84).

To be interviewed by a computer is one thing, but it is quite another to know that treatment will be determined by one. Although most patients are unaware of the degree to which technology is utilized to render diagnostic and treatment decisions, people are becoming more sophisticated in this respect. Moreover, they appear to be enthusiastic about this development. In an era where health care is frequently attacked as being highly dehumanized, expensive, and disorganized, only medicine's technological accomplishments have received widespread acclaim. Just as the public insists upon the greater availability of these services, it is reasonable to assume that as they become more aware of the superior ability of medical computers, they will not only accept, but actually demand, automated clinical care (52).

The emergence of a medic-computer model will depend on the public's acceptance of the machine as well as on their confidence in allied health professionals. Both patients and doctors are becoming more aware of the fact that physician's assistants and specially trained nurses can provide extensive and reliable clinical services. We are beginning to acknowledge that in the absence of extensive theoretical knowledge, nonphysicians are able to practice high-quality medicine (70).* As patients start to recognize the usefulness of paraprofessionals, they may not only feel more at ease with allied health personnel, but also may have less of a need to deify physicians.

The health-team model will be a necessary prelude to the emergence of a medic-computer model, a required testing ground for the eventual development of a Post-Physician Era. During the period in which this model will predominate, computer technology will have to be sufficiently developed and tested to pave the way for an automated decision making system. The public's experience with nurse-practitioners, nurse-clinicians, and physician's assistants will influence the likelihood of future patients accepting the medic.

Because the implementation of a health-team model is only in its initial stages, to conclude that patients definitely will accept medical care from allied health professionals would be premature. Nevertheless, evidence suggests that they would. Without any *major* difficulties nonphysicians have assumed primary clinical responsibilities in other nations for centuries (85). To the extent that allied health personnel have rendered clinical services in this country, patient acceptance has been favorable (71–72, 86–89). The only *widespread* use of paraprofessionals in the United States has been in the armed forces, where servicemen generally have been pleased by the care provided them by military corpsmen (70).

As physicians continue to withdraw from active patient care under a health-team model, the public will become less dependent upon doctors' services. As paraprofessionals increasingly utilize computers in providing clinical services (8, 52, 79, 86, 90), patients will become accustomed to receiving treatment from

---

* Of course, many doctors also practice medicine without a fundamental understanding of disease processes.

machine-assisted allied health personnel. The transition from a health-team to a medic-computer model could be a relatively smooth and undramatic one, unlikely to create an unusual amount of popular dissatisfaction or anxiety.

Although patients will accept a medic-computer model, will physicians do the same? I would propose that doctors will not only permit, but may actually *facilitate*, their own obsolescence. This hypothesis deserves careful examination, because professionals are hardly known to contribute to their own demise. To understand how physicians may disengage, however unwittingly, from the practice of medicine, one must examine the attitudes of doctors within a cultural and historical context.

In many respects physicians share with the general public the same ambivalence toward technology. Doctors cannot help but influence and be influenced by these prevailing social attitudes. To some extent, the physician's scientific background dovetails with cultural sentiments that are favorably disposed to the increasing deployment of technology. However, doctors are not immune to the outcries of the Neo-Luddites; so many contemporary physicians are reluctant to embrace the machine (91). Nevertheless, they, like everyone else will grow up in an increasingly automated world and progressively feel more at ease with the computer. Although computers currently play a limited role in medicine, many physicians fear that the machine will encroach upon their clinical activities. Almost every author who writes about the medical use of computers seems compelled to reassure the doctor that the machine will not replace him.

The pervasive concern among physicians that they could be rendered obsolete was illustrated in an editorial in *The New England Journal of Medicine*. This esteemed publication carried an article by Harold Sox *et al.* describing a protocol in which the logical diagnostic thought processes of a doctor were clearly delineated and specified so that they could be implemented by a physician's assistant. (The program, which is called an "algorithm," could be utilized by a computer.) Because the execution of this algorithm did not require an understanding of disease processes, almost anybody could implement it. All the user had to do was to follow a series of unambiguous step-by-step instructions to diagnose and treat a patient (8). An editorial writer in the same publication was offended by the possibilities that even a high school dropout could perform it. In a telling statement the author writes:

> No judgment whatsoever is expected from those guided along the algorithm's path; in fact, independent judgment must be rigorously avoided, for its exercise might well destroy the logic of the algorithm. Physician's-assistants who used independent judgment were rated by Sox as committing errors. Nor is the physician using an algorithm expected to think for himself.
>
> If understanding is unimportant and judgment is prohibited, what need is there for some knowledge of biochemistry, physiology, pharmacology, diagnostic interpretation or therapeutic rationale (92, p. 847)?*

The author does not object to the logic of the algorithm, nor even to its clinical utility. He is bothered (or frightened?) by the prospect that complex medical knowledge has been "reduced" to an easily followed set of directions. He goes on to ask, "What need is there, moreover, for an M.D. diploma, or even a college degree?" The answer to this question may be quite different from the one its author had implied. If algorithms can be developed and utilized by a physician's assistant or by a computer, the author may be right—what need is there for an M.D. diploma?

Not all physicians who discount the use of medical computers do so because they fear their own professional obsolescence. Some have based their objections upon more practical considerations. They cite the initial expense of the equipment, its lack of accessibility, the need for highly skilled computer personnel, and its failure to increase their clinical efficiency (9, 44, 93). Where these deficiencies have been overcome, physicians generally have been receptive to the use of medical computers (94–98). Another frequently heard objection to the machine is, as one doctor

* Reprinted, by permission from *The New England Journal of Medicine,* **288**: 847–848, 1973.

demurely put it, "I don't understand the damn things and therefore don't like them" (91). Undoubtedly, physicians issued similar pronouncements when EKGs, X-rays, and laboratory tests were first introduced, but as medical students learned to use these technical aids during their formal education, they readily accepted them as a routine part of clinical practice. Similarly, as student-physicians are trained to use medical computers, they will come to view them as being an indispensable tool for delivering patient care. Although contemporary doctors may be threatened by the computer, they may come to see the machine as an integral and necessary element in providing effective clinical services.

In the meantime a number of significant, albeit subtle, psychological trends suggest that physicians will abdicate their clinical role, not because they have to, but rather because they want to. In recent years an estimated 20 to 25 percent of all student doctors have felt estranged from medicine and its institutions. These alienated students have been "turned off" by what they feel is the stultifying and dehumanizing effect of clinical practice and medical education. They have chosen to invest a greater portion of their energies in political and, more recently aesthetic pursuits, hoping that these endeavors will help to fill a void they perceive as a result of their medical school experiences (99–101). This disenchantment with clinical medicine is not limited to student-physicians; many doctors wish to divest themselves of patient care responsibilities and to assume other types of medical activities. Fleeing from a seemingly unending onslaught of coughing, sneezing and whining kids, many harassed pediatricians are entering child psychiatry. For numerous reasons other practitioners are abdicating their clinical responsibilities to assume more challenging activities. For example, from 1963 to 1973 physicians' time devoted to patient care increased 19.6 percent; during the same interval time devoted to other professional endeavors increased 97 percent. (During this decade the number of doctors rose by 32.5 percent.) The most striking increase was in the field of administration, where the allocation of physicians' hours rose by 258.9 percent (37). Some doctors confess that although they had looked forward to medical practice, eventually this feeling of novelty gave way to a sense of monotony. The day-in-and-day-out routine of seeing patients, although financially advantageous, did not offer the kind of personal and intellectual satisfactions that they envisioned. As a result, many embarked upon investigatory, educational, or administrative careers. Of course, many contemporary physicians genuinely delight in providing patient care. However, from 1963 to 1973 the proportion of physicians engaged in patient care activities has declined by 10 percent, while the proportion of doctors performing medical research has increased by 92 percent (37). Obviously, a growing number of physicians appear driven to extend their knowledge of disease processes. As Kierkegaard observed, "Knowledge is an attitude, a passion; actually an illicit attitude. For the compulsion to know is just like dipsomania, erotomania, homicidal mania, in producing a character that is out of balance. It is not at all true that the scientist goes after truth. It goes after him. It is something he suffers from" (102, p. 329).

Another manifestation of the trend away from clinical practice is that recently American doctors have expressed a greater interest in allowing allied health personnel to perform duties formerly conducted solely by physicians. In a survey of 3,425 internists, the participants felt that paraprofessionals could handle many routine clinical responsibilities, such as routine history taking (60 percent), house calls (65 percent), patient instruction (70 percent), nursing home visits (43 percent), and the performance of Pap smears (34 percent) (103). The American Academy of Pediatrics found that over 70 percent of the 5,799 pediatricians sampled favored the use of allied health workers to gather selected elements of the history, and to counsel parents on child care, feeding, and development. More than 50 percent felt that paraprofessionals should make home visits and provide medical advice on minor clinical matters. A smaller number favored delegating well-child examinations (25 percent), sick-child examinations (20 percent), and newborn visits to maternity hospitals (32 percent) to allied health personnel (104). Although these surveys suggest that doctors are growing receptive to the *idea* that nonphysicians can and should assume some clinical responsibilities, they also show that doctors are hesitant about utilizing these individuals in their own practices. For example, these and other studies reveal that although 60 percent of doctors want additional help, only 30 percent of them would be inclined to employ paraprofessionals to provide that help (86, 105). This finding seems to reflect the cautious attitudes frequently held by physicians. The concept of utilizing nurse-clinicians, nurse-practitioners, and physician's assistants is relatively new to American medicine, and doctors are not known to leap into unfamiliar ventures. Nevertheless, where paraprofessionals have been tried, doctors have been pleased by their performance (70–72, 87, 106). As more physicians begin to appreciate the benefits that can accrue from the team approach, * the use of allied health personnel will undoubtedly accelerate. If so, paraprofessionals will usurp the doctor's role in providing many forms of patient care and they will do so with the active encouragement of physicians. As doctors continue to divest themselves of clinical responsibilities, paraprofessionals will be assuming many of the tasks previously performed by the medical profession. These coexisting trends would seem to meet the doctor's need to escape from the tedium of routine clinical practice, while simultaneously providing the allied health professional with the gratifying and challenging tasks of offering medical services. The transition from a physician-centered to a health-team model would satisfy all concerned.

The evolution from a health-team to a medic-computer model may occur for somewhat different reasons. In advocating the more extensive use of allied health professionals and computers for delivering clinical services, many have assumed that these developments would allow physicians to concentrate on either the more supportive or the more specialized aspects of patient care. However, doctors, with their extensive scientific training, would not seem to be eager to devote their major clinical efforts

---

* The team approach does present difficulties. For the sake of clarity, however, various aspects of these problems are discussed in Chapters 3, 5, and 7.

to providing emotional comfort to patients (52). They may prefer
to have nonphysicians, such as medics, assume these responsibilities. Simultaneously computers will be gathering histories
and rendering accurate clinical decisions, and it would be unlikely that doctors will acquire very much gratification from
executing more specialized medical tasks. Highly trained physicians will not be suited by temperament to perform tasks that
could be delivered more readily and more effectively by a medic
or by a computer. Because physicians are not going to *want* to do
something that a medic-computer symbiosis could do better, they
may actually facilitate the development of a medic-computer
model.

One of the factors that makes a future Post-Physician Era
difficult to envision is that it is difficult to imagine the future at
all. We can think and speculate about the future, even plan for
it, but somehow it still remains illusive. It lacks the concreteness
of the present. It appears suspended within a time capsule,
located somewhere between the reality of our lives and the
unreality of our dreams.

THE QUEST FOR MEDICAL HUMANISM.   Humanists decry
that our automated society is giving rise to a generation of
"technical giants and spiritual pygmies" (107, p. 101). They
maintain that advancing technology is generating a pervasive
sense of alienation. Unless we extricate ourselves from this
"cybernated nightmare," we shall soon become as inhuman as
the machines that dominate us. This assumption must be examined carefully, especially when viewed within a medical
context. These prophets of doom have suggested that the increased use of computers will further dehumanize the delivery of
clinical services. However, if one compares a physician-centered
to a medic-computer model, alternative conclusions may be
drawn.

A health care system that provides inferior medical services is
not humanistic. Despite our vast economic, technical, and human
resources, in a comparison of the 22 most industrialized countries

in the world, the United States ranks 15th in infant mortality and its life expectancies rate 19th for males and 6th for females (108).* Moreover, because our knowledge of disease processes is expanding exponentially, doctors are unable to keep abreast of current developments. They either deliver outmoded forms of medical treatment or provide only highly specialized services. Under a medic-computer model, the machine would be able to offer the most advanced level of available clinical decision making. A computer would not be limited by time, experience, and training as a physician is. An automated system could be updated frequently with information derived from the entire body of collected medical data. Unlike the doctor, the properly programmed computer would function around the clock, without making mistakes because it is tired, bored, irritable, or forgetful. Because the machine could provide the highest level of available clinical care, it would be unreasonable to attack its medical use from an ethical perspective.

A system of health care in which so many physicians are preoccupied with technical chores that they are unwilling or unable to meet the emotional needs of their patients is not humanistic. The problem of depersonalized medical care cannot be resolved successfully by simply deemphasizing the technical side of medical education and by augmenting the psychological skills of the doctor. Physicians must learn a vast amount of scientific information; without this knowledge the doctor cannot be distinguished from the quack. The acquisition and performance of skills has become so demanding that many doctors simply do not have the opportunity to provide emotional support (53). However, even if they did, physicians are not necessarily suited by temperament to concentrate on psychological issues (52). They generally are admitted

---

* Although important, the delivery of inferior medical services is not the only or even necessarily the major reason why the United States ranks so poorly on these commonly used indexes of a nation's health. Many other factors, such as the organization and the priorities of our health care system, are responsible for this unfortunate state of affairs (50, 53, 76, 109–110). In the following chapter I illustrate that the existence of a physician-centered model is responsible partially for the organizational difficulties and the faulty priorities in our health care system.

to medical schools because of their scientific expertise rather than because of their interpersonal skills (111–112). Not only do physicians have a predilection to focus on medicine's technical aspects, but out of necessity this tendency is fostered throughout their training (113). Furthermore, the belief that an educational system can change a scientifically oriented student into a psychologically sensitive physician remains to be seen. An individual's ability to relate to people has been formed throughout his premedical years and cannot readily be transformed by the issuance of moral imperatives by humanistically inclined professors. A medic could be chosen primarily because of his experience and skill in interpersonal relations. Because the computer would perform most of the technical aspects of patient care, the medic would be free to concentrate almost exclusively on the emotional side of clinical medicine. Without the albatross of having to learn and implement extensive technical chores, the medic would be able to emulate Roger Chillingsworth, the physician in *The Scarlet Letter*. As Nathaniel Hawthorne wrote of him, "He deemed it essential, it would seem, to know the man before attempting to do him good."

A system of medical care that is unavailable to millions of Americans is not humanistic. More than anyone else the inadequacies of the health system afflict the poor; among the poor, Blacks, Puerto Ricans, Chicanos, and American Indians are the most affected. Because of inadequate housing, nutrition, sanitation, education, and medical care, the disadvantaged tend to be condemned to poor health from conception to death. The infant mortality rate is approximately 44 percent higher for nonwhites, who live 6.4 years less than whites (37). Moreover, our present physician-centered model fails to provide health services to many rural communities as well as to urban ghettos. For example, in the mid-Atlantic states there is one doctor for every 585 individuals; in the East South Central portion of the United States there is one doctor for every 1,124 citizens (108). There are 134 counties in 36 states without a single physician, and hundreds more with only one or two practitioners. In desperation many of these communities launch extravagant campaigns, with billboards and medical journal advertisements to lure physicians. Frequently they offer a doctor a suite of rent-free offices, a splendid house, and a guaranteed income (110). But even these efforts fail to produce the desired results.

So critical is the doctor shortage that many communities and hospitals are forced to recruit foreign physicians who often have major linguistic and medical limitations. Approximately one-fifth of the doctors practicing in the United States are graduates of foreign medical schools, and the trend has been going upward. In 1972, the last year for which statistics are available, 7,943 American graduates and 6,661 foreign medical graduates were licensed in the United States (114). Although some of these students are American-born, nearly 33 percent of newly licensed doctors in this country each year are foreign nationals (115). That the richest country in the world depletes the scarce medical resources of other nations to compensate for its own deficiencies is embarrassing, if not unconscionable. Some critics have maintained that stronger government interventions will lead to a more equitable distribution of physicians (108). However, even in the Soviet Union, where the government has extensive control over the distribution of physicians, getting doctors to practice in remote areas is still difficult (116).

Others have claimed that the problem of unavailable medical care is not caused primarily by a maldistribution of physicians, but results from an inadequate number of doctors (53, 108, 117). According to the National Institute of Health's Health Manpower Bureau, in 1970 there was an estimated shortage of 48,000 physicians in the United States alone (118). Many believe the answer to this dilemma lies in training more doctors (108), but this would only be a stopgap measure (52, 119). In the Soviet Union, where a more favorable doctor–patient ratio exists than in the United States (1:375 to 1:582), they still have difficulties providing care to many isolated communities (116).

Although the implementation of comprehensive national health insurance, the education of an increasing number of doctors, and the more equitable distribution of physicians may help to alleviate the health care crisis, these developments, even if they do occur, will not solve the fundamental dilemma of unavailable medical personnel. As long as we perpetuate a physician-centered model, these problems will persist. But a medic-computer model could surpass a physician-centered model by offering medical care to those who presently are denied it. Because the services of a computer can be transmitted via telephone lines, even the most remote areas of the country could have access to automated medical decision making. At the same time, assuming medics will distribute themselves as nurses have, they would be more likely to practice in locations that presently lack physicians. Furthermore, unlike doctors, medics could be trained within a relatively brief period of time, and therefore, a significantly greater pool of medics would be available to assume clinical responsibilities.

A health care system in which physicians treat minority group members with an inadequate understanding of their mores, attitudes, and problems is not humanistic. A physician-centered model is inherently discriminatory. It denies access to the medical profession of minority group physicians who would be more likely than their middle class colleagues to understand the life problems and communication styles of their economically deprived patients (31, 124). The enormous costs of receiving extensive professional training, the lack of persistent cultural and parental encouragement (120), racism, and inadequate educational opportunities prior to entering medical school have all contributed to the unfortunate situation in which the vast majority of doctors come from the white middle class. Consequently, the medical profession and the society is denied the stimulation and enrichment that cultural and racial diversity could provide (116). Despite the moderately successful efforts of medical schools in recent years to expand the number of minority groups students,* these attempts will be unlikely to compensate substantially for the extensive

---

* In 1973, although Black, Chicano, and Hispanic Americans constituted 15.8 percent of the population (37), they represented only 8.8 percent of first-year medical students (121). Although this is an improvement from 1968 when they were less than 3 percent of the nation's freshman medical school class (122), I am afraid that the declining social consciousness of the 1970s may induce medical schools to relax their efforts at recruiting minority students.

economic, educational, and social disadvantages that many experts believe will increasingly plague the lower classes in the future (123).

The relatively brief education required to train the medic would enhance the inclusion of minority group members in the overall pool of medical manpower. Just as doctors tend to practice where their own ethnic group resides (125), Black, Chicano, Hispanic and American Indian medics also would be more likely to practice among their own groups. Furthermore, unlike the prejudicial attitudes of some physicians, computers could render medical decisions without racial bias. A medic-computer model could enhance the quality and dignity of health care delivered to minority groups.

A health care system in which the rigorous demands and mechanized nature of providing patient care engenders a profound sense of dissatisfaction among physicians is not humanistic. Their relatively high divorce and suicide rate (126) suggests that the practice of medicine may be "hazardous to their health." Whereas the doctor once derived considerable gratification from the invigorating intellectual challenges of rendering accurate diagnostic and treatment decisions, the increasing role of medical computers will only augment the discontent experienced by many practicing physicians. There is little reason for doctors to execute tasks that a computer could do better. As A. M. Uttley observed, "Machines will slowly take over from men all the tedious thinking which yet must be done without error; all the sorting and checking and counting and repetitive calculation which, frankly, makes machines of us" (21, p. 22). In a moment of candor one medical student told me, "Whenever I take a history from a patient *I* begin to feel like a computer." Undoubtedly, the majority of his classmates would not share this extreme viewpoint. Nevertheless, a significant number of student-physicians identify with his sense of being mechanized by the practice of medicine (99–101).

Under a medic-computer model those individuals who receive gratification from relating to patients will have the opportunity to do so as a medic, without being sidetracked by having to perform extensive technical procedures. Similarly, those individuals who enjoy the challenges of medical research, education, or administration would be able to devote themselves fully to these endeavors. The obsolescence of the physician will not contribute to the obsolescence of man. Instead the actualization of a Post-Physician Era will allow would-be doctors to pursue those careers that would bring them maximum satisfaction.

For all of these reasons, I am unable to agree with those who, at least within a medical context, equate automation with dehumanization. As a physician, I am thankful for the advances in technology that have permitted me to alleviate suffering and to cure disease. As a patient, I have been grateful for those mechanized "monsters," such as EKGs and automated laboratories, that in large measure have restored my health. To deny myself or others the advantages of these products of technology to satisfy some technophobic whim, would be cruel and inhumane. Regardless of how well-intentioned, those who advocate a moratorium on the use of medical technology would thwart man's humanistic desire for a healthier and more vital populace (128).

SUMMARY. From a technical, economic, social, psychohistorical and humanistic perspective, we no longer will have to adhere to the myth of physician necessity. Moreover, I cannot agree with the numerous authors who claim that our ailing health care system can be cured largely by modifying the economic, educational, or organizational context of medical practice (6, 50, 53, 70, 109–110, 119, 128–134). Instead, I am suggesting that our current health crisis will continue until we recognize that doctors themselves, regardless of their sincerity, education, or skill, are to a great extent the essence of the problem. Before the emergence of advanced technology we had to rely upon physicians; no other viable alternatives existed. However, computers afford us a new opportunity to rectify the deficiencies of contemporary medicine. If we are to plan for the future, we must think seriously about the innovative use of these technological resources.

NOTES

1. Boyle, J. A., and J. A. Anderson (1968). "Computer Diagnosis: Clinical Aspects." *British Medical Journal*, 24:224–229.

2. Sterling, T. D., J. Nickson, and S. V. Pollack (1966). "Is Medical Diagnosis A General Computer Problem?" *Journal of the American Medical Association*, 198:191–196.

3. Eisenberg, H. (1973). "1978: Art Vs. Science." *Medical Economics*, 50 (22):20–34.

4. Freidson, E. (1972). *Profession of Medicine: A Study of the Sociology of Applied Knowledge.* New York: Dodd, Mead.

5. Norwood, W. F. (1970). "Medical Education in the United States Before 1900." In C. D. O'Malley (ed.), *The History of Medical Education.* Berkeley: University of California Press. Pp. 463–499.

6. Rutstein, D. D. (1967). *The Coming Revolution in Medicine.* Cambridge: M.I.T. Press.

7. Barry, M. J. (1968). "Non-Neurotic Neurotics." *Postgraduate Medicine*, 43(4):87–91.

8. Sox, H. C., Jr., C. H. Sox, R. K. Tompkins (1973). "The Training of Physician's Assistants: The Use of A Clinical Algorithm System for Patient Care, Audit of Performance and Education." *New England Journal of Medicine*, 288:818–824.

9. Sidel, V. W. (1971). "New Technologies and the Practice of Medicine." In E. Mendelsohn, J. P. Swazey, and I. Taviss (eds.), *Human Aspects of Biomedical Innovation.* Cambridge: Harvard University Press. Pp. 131–155.

10. Wortman, P. M. (1972). "Medical Diagnosis: An Information-Processing Approach." *Computers and Biomedical Research*, 5:315–328.

11. Mayne, J. G., W. Weksel, and P. N. Sholtz (1968). "Toward Automating the Medical History." *Mayo Clinic Proceedings*, 43(1):1–25.

12. Payne, L. C. (1964). "The Role of the Computer in Refining Diagnosis." *Lancet*, 2:32–35.

13. Greist, J. H., D. H. Gustafson, F. F. Stauss, G. L. Rowse, T. P. Laughren, and J. A. Chiles (1973). "A Computer Interview for Suicide-Risk Prediction." *American Journal of Psychiatry*, 130:1327–1332.

14. Barnett, G. O. (1968). "Computers in Patient Care." *New England Journal of Medicine*, 279:1321–1327.

15. Warner, H. R., C. M. Olmsted, and B. D. Rutherford (1972). "HELP— A Program for Medical Decision-Making." *Computers and Biomedical Research*, 5(1):65–74.

16. Kemeny, J. G. (1972). *Man and the Computer.* New York: Scribner's.

17. Overall, J. E., and C. M. Williams (1963). "Conditional Probability Program for Diagnosis of Thyroid Function." *Journal of the American Medical Association*, 183:307–313.

18. Dumont, M. P. (1972). "The Computer Sees the Truth But Waits: The Junkie As Political Enemy: II." *American Journal*, 1(2):7.

19. Hall, G. H. (1967). "The Clinical Application of Bayes' Theorem." *Lancet*, 2(Part I):555–557.

20. Ledley, R. S. (1966). "Computer Aids to Medical Diagnosis." *Journal of the American Medical Association*, 196:933-943.

21. Fink, D. G. (1966). *Computers and the Human Mind.* Garden City, N. J.: Doubleday.

22. Feinberg, G. (1969). *The Prometheus Project: Mankind's Search for Long-Range Goals.* Garden City, N. J.: Doubleday.

23. Sletten, I. W., H. Altman, G. A. Ulett (1971). "Routine Diagnosis by Computer." *American Journal of Psychiatry*, 127:1147–1152.

24. Zarnstorff, W. C., W. R. Hendee, and P. L. Carson (eds.) (1972). *Application of Optical Instrumentation in Medicine.* Chicago: Society of Photo-Optical Instrumentation Engineers.

25. Brodman, K., A. J. Van Woerkman, A. J. Erdmann, Jr., and L. S. Goldstein (1959). "Interpretation of Symptoms With A Data-Processing Machine." *Archives of Internal Medicine*, 103:776–782.

26. Toronto, A. F., L. G. Veasey, and H. R. Warner (1963). "Evaluation of A Computer Program for Diagnosis of Congenital Heart Disease." *Progress in Cardiovascular Diseases*, 5:362–377.

27. Eden, M. (1969). "Computers in Biomedicine-II." In J. F. Dickson III, and J. H. U. Brown (eds.), *Future Goals of Engineering in Biology and Medicine.* New York: Academic. Pp. 216–221.

28. Spitzer R. L., J. Endicott, J. Cohen, and J. L. Fleiss (1974). "Constraints on the Validity of Computer Diagnosis." *Archives of General Psychiatry*, 31: 197–203.

29. Pipberger, H. V., and J. Cornfield (1973). "What ECG Computer Program to Choose for Clinical Application: The Need for Consumer Protection." *Circulation*, 47:918–920.

30. Panzetta, A. F. (1974). "Toward A Scientific Psychiatric Nosology: Conceptual and Pragmatic Issues." *Archives of General Psychiatry*, 30:154–161.

31. Mechanic, D. (1968). *Medical Sociology: A Selective View.* New York: Free Press.

32. Kahn, H., and A. J. Wiener (1967). *Toward the Year 2000: A Framework for Speculation.* New York: Macmillan.

33. Gottlieb, G. L., R. F. Beers, Jr., C. Bernecker, and M. Samter (1972). "An Approach to Automation of Medical Interviews." *Computers and Biomedical Research*, 5:99–107.

34. Heyman, A. (1966). "Spirochetal Diseases." In T. R. Harrison, R. D. Adams, I. L. Bennett, Jr., W. H. Resnick, G. W. Thorn, and M. M. Wintrobe (eds.), *Principles of Internal Medicine.* New York: McGraw-Hill. Pp. 1628–1641.

35. Berkley, C. (ed.) (1971). *Automatic Multiphasic Health Testing*. New York: Engineering Foundation.

36. Goldberg, M., S. B. Green, M. L. Moss, C. B. Marbach, and D. Garfinkel (1973). "Computer-Based Instruction and Diagnosis of Acid-Base Disorders." *Journal of the American Medical Association*, 223:269–275.

37. Eisenberg, B. S. and P. Aherne (eds.) (1974). *Socioeconomic Issues of Health '74*. Chicago: American Medical Association.

38. Toffler, A. (1971). *Future Shock*. New York: Bantam.

39. Samuel, A. L. (1959). "Some Studies in Machine Learning Using the Game of Checkers." *IBM Journal of Research and Development*, 3:210–229.

40. Samuel, A. L. (1967). "Some Studies in Machine Learning Using the Game of Checkers. II—Recent Progress." *IBM Journal of Research and Development*, 11:601–617.

41. Stehling, K. R. (1972). *Computers and You*. New York: New American Library.

42. Mesthene, E. G. (1970). *Technological Change: Its Impact on Man and Society*. New York: New American Library.

43. Taviss, I. (1971). "Problems in the Social Control of Biomedical Science and Technology." In E. Mendelsohn, J. P. Swazey, and I. Taviss (eds.), *Human Aspects of Biomedical Innovation*. Cambridge: Harvard University Press. Pp. 3–45.

44. Baird, H. W., and J. M. Garfunkel (1965). "Electronic Data Processing of Medical Records." *New England Journal of Medicine*, 272:1211–1215.

45. Martin, J., and A. R. D. Norman (1970). *The Computerized Society*. Englewood Cliffs, N. J.: Prentice-Hall.

46. Sarnoff, D. (1966). "No Life Untouched." *Saturday Review*, 49(30):21–22.

47. Culliton, B. J. (1974). "Medical Education: Institute Puts A Price on Doctors' Heads." *Science*, 183(4131):1272–1274.

48. *Medical World News* (1973). "The Rising Cost of Medical Education," 14(9):4.

49. Oppenheim. G. (1973). "1978: Work Vs. Leisure." *Medical Economics*, 50(22):162–182.

50. Greenberg, S. (1971). *The Quality of Mercy: A Report on the Critical Condition of Hospital and Medical Care in America*. New York: Atheneum.

51. Field, M. G. (1973). "The Health System and the Social System." Paper delivered at the Conference on Medical Sociology in Warsaw, August 20–25.

52. Schwartz, W. B. (1970). "Medicine and the Computer: The Promise and Problems of Change." *New England Journal of Medicine*, 283:1257–1264.

53. Mechanic, D. (1972). *Public Expectations and Health Care: Essays on the Changing Organization of Health Services*. New York: Wiley-Interscience.

54. Harvard University Program on Technology and Society (1968). *Implications of Biomedical Technology*, Research Review No. 1. Cambridge.

55. *Medical World News* (1969). "Who Will Lead the AMA . . . and Where?" 10(27):24–32.

56. Altman, L. K. (1975). "A.M.A. Approves $140 Increase in Dues." *New York Times*, June 19. P. 32.

57. Maxmen, J. S. (1970). "On Joining the AMA." *Medical Opinion and Review*, 6(9):50–57.

58. Fuchs, V. R. (1970). "Can the Traditional Practice of Medicine Survive?" *Archives of Internal Medicine*, 125:154–156.

59. Freed, R. N. (1967). "Legal Aspects of Computer Use in Medicine." *Law and Contemporary Problems*, 32:674–706.

60. Ellul, J. (1964). *The Technological Society*. New York: Vintage.

61. Reich, C. A. (1970). *The Greening of America: How the Youth Revolution Is Trying to Make America Livable*. New York: Random House.

62. Roszak, T. (1968). *The Making of the Counter Culture: Reflections on the Technocratic Society and Its Youthful Opposition*. Garden City, N. J.: Doubleday.

63. Branscomb, L. M. (1971). "Why People Fear Technology." *The Futurist*, 5:232.

64. de Bono, E. (1971). "Technology Today." In E. de Bonò (ed.), *Technology Today*. London: Routledge & Kegan Paul. Pp. 1–36.

65. Lidz, T. (1968). *The Person: His Development Throughout the Life Cycle*. New York: Basic Books.

66. Erikson, E. H. (1963). *Childhood and Society*. New York: Norton.

67. Diebold, J. (1970). *Man & the Computer: Technology as an Agent of Social Change*. New York: Avon.

68. Field, M. G. (1971). "The Health Care System of Industrial Society: The Disappearance of the General Practitioner and Some Implications." In E. Mendelsohn, J. P. Swazey, and I. Taviss (eds.), *Human Aspects of Biomedical Innovation*. Cambridge: Harvard University Press. Pp. 156–180.

69. Stead, E. A., Jr. (1973). "Family Practice: One View." In J. Graves (ed.), *The Future of Medical Education*. Durham, N. C.: Duke University Press. Pp. 143–154.

70. Sadler, A. M. Jr., B. L. Sadler, and A. A. Bliss (1972). *The Physician's Assistant: Today and Tomorrow*. New Haven: Yale University Press.

71. Lohrenz, F. N. (1971). "The Marshfield Clinic Physician-Assistant Concept." *New England Journal of Medicine*, 284:301–304.

72. Rogers, K. D., M. Mally, F. L. Marcus (1968). "A General Medical Practice Using Nonphysician Personnel." *Journal of the American Medical Association*, 206:1753–1757.

73. Strauss, M. B. (ed.) (1968). *Familiar Medical Quotations*. Boston: Little, Brown.

74. Erikson. E. H. (1974). *Dimensions of A New Identity: The 1973 Jefferson Lectures in the Humanities*. New York: Norton.

75. Hooker, W. (1844). *Dissertation on the Respect Due to the Medical Profession*

and the Reasons That It Is Not Awarded by the Community. Norwich, Conn.: J. G. Cooley.

76. Dubos, R. (1965). Man Adapting. New Haven: Yale University Press.

77. Slack, W. V., and C. W. Slack (1972). "Patient-Computer Dialogue." New England Journal of Medicine, 286:1304–1309.

78. Coddington, R. D., and T. L. King (1972). "Automated History Taking in Child Psychiatry." American Journal of Psychiatry, 129:276–282.

79. Grossman, J. H., G. O. Barnett, M. T. McGuire, and D. B. Swedlow (1971). "Evaluation of Computer-Acquired Patient Histories." Journal of the American Medical Association, 215:1286–1291.

80. Slack, W. V., G. P. Hicks, C. E. Reed, and L. J. Van Cura (1966). "A Computer-Based Medical-History System." New England Journal of Medicine, 274:194–198.

81. Greist, J. H., L. J. Van Cura, and N. P. Kneppreth (1973). "A Computer Interview for Emergency Room Patients." Computers and Biomedical Research, 6:257–265.

82. Greist, J. H., M. H. Klein, and L. J. Van Cura (1973). "A Computer Interview for Psychiatric Patient Target Symptoms." Archives of General Psychiatry, 29:247–253.

83. Haessler, H. A. (1971). "The Interactive, Self-Administered Medical History." In C. Berkley (ed.), Automated Multiphasic Health Testing. New York: Engineering Foundation. Pp. 276–286.

84. Korsch, B. M., and V. F. Neguete (1972). "Doctor-Patient Communication." Scientific American, 227(2): 66–74.

85. Kadish, J., and J. W. Long (1970). "The Training of Physician Assistants: Status and Issues," Journal of the American Medical Association, 212: 1047–1051.

86. Carlson, C. L., and G. T. Athelstan (1970). "The Physician's Assistant: Versions and Diversions of A Promising Concept." Journal of the American Medical Association, 214:1855–1861.

87. Silver, H. K., and P. A. McAtee (1972). "Who Will Provide More Health Care?—II." Medical Tribune, 13(48):5.

88. Litman, T. J. (1972). "Public Perceptions of the Physicians' Assistant— A Survey of the Attitudes and Opinions of Rural Iowa and Minnesota Residents." American Journal of Public Health. 62:343–346.

89. Nelson, E. C., A. R. Jacobs, and K. G. Johnson (1974). "Patients' Acceptance of Physician's Assistants." Journal of the American Medical Association, 228:63–67.

90. Collen, M. F. (1966). "Periodic Health Examinations Using an Automated Multitest Laboratory." Journal of the American Medical Association, 195:830–833.

91. Scott, B. (1971). "What Physicians Think about Computers, Transplants and the 'PA.' " Medical Opinion and Review, 7(8):46–48.

92. Ingelfinger, F. J. (1973). "Algorithms, Anyone?" *New England Journal of Medicine*, 288:847–848.

93. Caceres, C. A. (1969). "Computers in Biomedicine-I." In J. F. Dickson III, and J. H. U. Brown (eds.), *Future Goals of Engineering and Biology in Medicine*. New York: Academic. Pp. 206–215.

94. Menn, S. J., G. O. Barnett, D. Schmechel, W. D. Owens, and H. Pontoppidan (1973). "A Computer Program to Assist in the Care of Acute Respiratory Failure." *Journal of the American Medical Association*, 223: 308–312.

95. Greist, J. H. (1973). Personal Communication, April 6.

96. Greenes, R. A., G. O. Barnett, S. W. Klein, A. Robbins, and R. E. Prior (1970). "Recording, Retrieval, and Review of Medical Data by Physician-Computer Interaction." *New England Journal of Medicine*, 282:307–315.

97. Slack, W. V., B. M. Peckham, L. J. Van Cura, and W. F. Carr (1967). "A Computer-Based Physical Examination System." *Journal of the American Medical Association*, 200:224–228.

98. *Computers and Medicine* (1973). "MIS-1 After A Full Year's Operation—Pros & Cons," 2(6):1, 2 & 4.

99. Maxmen, J. S. (1971). "Medical Student Radicals: Conflict and Resolution." *American Journal of Psychiatry*, 127:1211–1215.

100. Maxmen, J. S. (1974). "The Alienated Medical Student: From Activism to Privatism." *Pharos*, 37:90–95.

101. Schwartz, A. H., and A. E. Slaby (1971). "Adjustment and Fantasy in Medical Students." *American Journal of Psychiatry*, 128:85–89.

102. Wilkins, M. H. F. (1972). "Possible Ways to Rebuild Science." In W. Fuller (ed.), *The Biological Revolution: Social Good or Social Evil?* Garden City, N. J.: Doubleday. Pp. 322–330.

103. Riddick, F. A., Jr., J. B. Bryan, M. I. Gershenson, and A. C. Costello (1971). "Use of Allied Health Professionals in Internists' Offices: Current Practices and Physicians' Attitudes." *Archives of Internal Medicine*, 127: 924–931.

104. Yankauer, A., J. P. Connelly, and J. J. Feldman (1970). "Pediatric Practice in the United States: With Special Attention to Utilization of Allied Health Worker Services." *Pediatrics*, 45:521–554.

105. Todd, M. C., and D. F. Foy (1972). "Current Status of the Physician's Assistant and Related Issues." *Journal of the American Medical Association*, 220:1714–1720.

106. *Journal of the American Medical Association* (1970). "Physician's Assistant or Assistant Physician?" 212:313.

107. MacEachen, A. J. (1972). "It Is Time to Humanize Technology." In R. Theobald (ed.), *Futures Conditional*. Indianapolis: Bobbs-Merrill. Pp. 98–112.

108. Carnegie Commission on Higher Education (1970). *Higher Education and*

the *Nation's Health: Policies for Medical and Dental Education.* New York: McGraw-Hill.

109. Chase, A. (1971). *The Biological Imperatives: Health, Politics, and Human Survival.* Baltimore: Penguin.

110. Ribicoff, A., and P. Danaceau (1973). *The American Medical Machine.* New York: Harrow.

111. Crowley, L. G., B. W. Nelson, and L. Aronow (1972). "How Stanford Selects New Medical Students." *Stanford M. D.*, 11(4):15–19.

112. Bradford, W. D. (1973). "Requirements for Admission to Medical School." In J. Graves (ed.), *The Future of Medical Education.* Durham, N. C.: Duke University Press. Pp. 53–69.

113. Eron, L. D. (1955). "Effect of Medical Education on Medical Students' Attitudes." *Journal of Medical Education*, 30:559–566.

114. *AAMC Education News* (1974). "AAMC Task Force on Foreign Graduates Places New Demands Upon MD Schools, Calls for Uniform Admission Standard." 1(5):1, 6.

115. National Board of Medical Examiners (1973). *Evaluation in the Continuum of Medical Education: Report of the Committee on Goals and Priorities.* Philadelphia: National Board of Medical Examiners.

116. Cherkasky, M. (1973). "Medical Education and Practice—Circa 1985." In J. Graves (ed.), *The Future of Medical Education.* Durham, N. C.: Duke University Press. Pp. 3–26.

117. Coggeshall, L. T. (1965). *Planning for Medical Progress Through Education.* Evanston, Ill.: Association of American Medical Colleges.

118. *American Medical News* (1970). "Health Manpower Shortages," 13(30):6.

119. Fuchs, V. R. (1975). "Another Case of the Whooping Crane?" *Prism*, 3(4):50–52.

120. Hall, O. (1958). "The Stages of A Medical Career." In E. G. Jaco (ed.), *Patients, Physicians and Illness.* Glencoe, Ill.: Free Press. Pp. 289–300.

121. Dubé, W. F. (1974). "U.S. Medical School Enrollment, 1969–70 through 1973–74." *Journal of Medical Education*, 49:302–307.

122. Dubé, W. F. (1973). "U.S. Medical Student Enrollments, 1968–1969 through 1972–1973." *Journal of Medical Education*, 48:293–297.

123. Miller, S. M., and P. A. Roby (1970). *The Future of Inequality.* New York: Basic Books.

124. Grier, W. H., and P. M. Cobbs (1968). *Black Rage.* New York: Basic Books.

125. Lieberson, S. (1958). "Ethnic Groups and the Practice of Medicine." *American Sociological Review*, 23:542–549.

126. Rose, K. D., and I. Rosow (1973). "Physicians Who Kill Themselves." *Archives of General Psychiatry*, 29:800–805.

127. Maxmen, J. S. (1973). "Goodbye, Dr. Welby." *Social Policy*, 3(4 & 5): 97–106.

128. Mendelsohn, E., J. P. Swazey, and I. Taviss (eds.) (1971). *Human Aspects of Biomedical Innovation.* Cambridge: Harvard University Press.

129. Graves, J. (ed.) (1973). *The Future of Medical Education*. Durham, N. C.: Duke University Press.

130. Kennedy, E. M. (1972). *In Critical Condition: The Crisis in America's Health Care*. New York: Simon and Schuster.

131. Ehrenreich, B., and J. Ehrenreich (1970). *The American Health Empire: Power, Profits, and Politics. A Report from the Health Policy Advisory Center (Health-PAC)*. New York: Random House.

132. Edwards, M. H. (1972). *Hazardous to Your Health: A New Look at the "Health Care Crisis" in America*. New Rochelle, N. Y.: Arlington House.

133. Tunley, R. (1966). *The American Health Scandal*. New York: Harper & Row.

134. Gerber, A. (1971). *The Gerber Report: The Shocking State of American Medical Care and What Must Be Done About It*. New York: McKay.

3

THE NEW MEDICAL
ORDER _____

Despite its numerous advantages, a Post-Physician Era will not become a medical utopia. Illness, Kafkaesque bureaucracies, inadequate continuity of care, impersonal practitioners, and violations of confidentiality may continue to disturb patients. Improper priorities, fiscal problems, widespread resistance to organizational restructuring, consumer demands, and political pressures may continue to plague administrators. Malpractice suits, government interventions, and legal restrictions may continue to harass health care personnel. Although these problems will persist, they are not unmanageable. Theoretically, the judicious use of organizational principles could ameliorate these dilemmas, just as the judicious use of medical technology could improve clinical decision making. Unfortunately, what is theoretically possible is not always pragmatically obtainable. For those who are engaged in the politics of change inevitably confront the psychology of resistance.

Although understandable, it is ironic that in the most protean of civilizations we continue to be unsettled by the specter of social change. I say "understandable" because the formation of our personal identities is dependent upon the existence of stable cultural values and institutions (1). Our identities are threatened by living in a nation where the only constant is change and the only tradition is transcience. Out of desperation we instinctively seek to ignore, deny, or even escape from the realities of a perpetually evolving society (2). Change is inevitable, and escape is no solution. Although we may flee from the future, we cannot prevent it. We can prepare for the future, so the world of tomorrow need not be so uncertain as the world of today.

Although some critics view social planning as the dangerous adventurism of an impersonal elite (3), such planning will be necessary if we are to minimize the difficulties enumerated in the opening paragraph of this chapter. Therefore, the important question is not if we should plan but how we should plan. The increasing utilization of computers and paraprofessionals will have a significant impact upon the overall health care system. Restructuring the organization of the health care system will affect enormously the introduction and operations of a medic-computer model. To avoid the chaos that could ensue from these anticipated developments we must design an effective organizational structure for the implementation and execution of a medic-computer model. How successfully we accomplish these objectives may determine if the New Medical Order becomes a humanitarian advance or a technological nightmare.

MAJOR ORGANIZATIONAL ISSUES. Numerous problems could be examined when discussing the organizational structure of any health care system, whether past, present, or future. Although the fundamental issues will remain the same, the changing nature of medical care may add new dimensions and offer novel solutions to these perennial concerns.

Control of the System. The group whose opinions and behavior ultimately determine the structure and function of the health care system control the system. No single group currently possesses *complete* hegemony; consumers, government officials, allied health professionals, labor unions, insurance companies, and doctors exercise varying degrees of authority. Although physicians represent only 10 percent of the health workers in the United States (4), more than anyone else they define and control the basic organizational pattern of medical services. This power derives from their specialized training, consumer demand, public prestige, considerable autonomy, and authority over the activities of the other health occupations (5–6). By virtue of maintaining primary control over the organization and structure of the medical care system, they also determine the conditions of clinical practice. Generally speaking, physicians operate under what economist Victor Fuchs calls the "technologic imperative." By this he means that most doctors feel that ethical medical practice requires them to use whatever technology is available to benefit their patients. Undoubtedly, this belief is shared by the general public. However, as Fuchs observes, in a society with limited human and fiscal health resources, the provision of optimal services to one segment of the population necessitates that the rest of the citizenry receive substandard care (7).

Most physicians define their primary responsibility as serving the needs of individual patients rather than of society as a whole. Under a system where patients choose their physician, doctors naturally feel beholden to the individual contracting their services. Moreover, a broad social perspective is difficult when doctors function in a one-to-one relationship with their clients in the privacy of their offices (8). And finally, it would be absurd to expect physicians to say to a patient, "I'm sorry, but despite the seriousness of your problem, I am not going to do everything possible to help you because that would prevent me from devoting myself to the overall health needs of the nation."

Although some authors would suggest that physicians should provide the greatest good for the greatest number (6), this expectation is unrealistic, given the psychological and economic realities of clinical practice under a physician-centered model. As long as doctors control the conditions of clinical work in a society with limited medical resources, the greatest good for the greatest

number will never be the top priority of our health care system. *
This priority can materialize only when the federal government
gains control over the structure and organization of our health care
system. The medical profession's rhetoric about the "sanctity of
the doctor-patient relationship" is often used as a guise under
which physicians hope to forestall government control over clinical
practice. However, before one condemns physicians for so
vehemently defending their own self-interest, we should remember that they are no different than other professionals, such as
attorneys and businessmen, who equally resent the government
controlling the conditions of their work.

Most observers believe that future government officials will
be restrained in restructuring the health care system to accommodate to the wishes of the medical profession. As sociologist David
Mechanic points out, "Although it is possible to construct ideal
models of what medical care should be, the types of medical care
programs that will evolve in the future will be of the same cloth
that presently exists" (6, p. 62). His view is correct as long as
doctors are the principal providers of clinical services. Even under
a health-team model physicians would continue to have considerable authority, and therefore, they would still exercise enormous control over the delivery of medical care. However, with the
advent of a medic-computer model, government will not be forced
to structure the health care system to meet the demands of the
medical profession. Because tomorrow's medics will have less
political power than today's doctors, a Post-Physician Era will
afford consumers a greater opportunity to control the operations
and structure of the health care system. The ramifications of this
change could be extensive; if doctors no longer exert primary control over the conditions of clinical practice, all of the remaining
organizational issues I shall raise will be affected.

Establishing Priorities. Priorities must be set within a health
care system of limited fiscal, technological, and human resources.

_____

* Of course one could debate if it ought to be the top priority.

Because doctors primarily control the system, especially in the United States, established priorities more often reflect the desires and interests of the medical profession than they do the health needs of the nation. For example, in Chapter 1 I noted how this situation has led to an excessive number of operations being performed in this country. Conversely, evidence indicates that prenatal and postnatal care of pregnant mothers and newborn children would significantly reduce morbidity and mortality rates. Yet these relatively inexpensive forms of care are frequently unavailable (6). In addition, in establishing priorities as to how physicians will be distributed, professional self-interest takes precedence over genuine public need. A 1972 survey conducted by the American Medical Association and the Rand Corporation revealed that the reasons doctors gave for deciding where they would practice included factors such as climate, per capita income of the area, degree of urbanization, availability of hospital beds, incomes of physicians in the community, the presence of a medical school, and the existence of nearby recreational and sports facilities (4). Nowhere in the survey did it show that the unmet health requirements of the populace was a determining variable. As long as physicians control the conditions of clinical practice, more justifiable medical priorities will hardly be implemented.

Assuming that under a medic-computer model the government would primarily control the operations of the health care system, more sensible and equitable priorities could be determined and executed. I do not wish to imply that setting priorities in a Post-Physician Era will be an easy task. It will still be a complex endeavor involving economic, scientific, humanitarian, and especially political considerations. The establishment of priorities will have to accommodate to the interests of consumers, health workers, and politicians. Government officials will need to consult researchers to help themselves distinguish between useful and wasteful medical interventions. And finally, inequalities in the delivery of health care services will have to be identified and rectified. Although establishing equitable medical priorities will continue to be difficult, this task will be accomplished more successfully in a society in which doctors do not exercise undue influence.

Standards of Care.   Because all medical procedures vary in their efficacy, availability, and costs, an important issue confronting any health care system is *who* decides which diagnostic and treatment measures ought to be utilized. Under a physician-centered model doctors make these determinations. However, as previously mentioned, these decisions frequently leave much to be desired. Some physicians perform unnecessary and at times even dangerous procedures for either personal profit or professional prestige. Others may do so out of ignorance or to avoid a malpractice suit. Because doctors cherish their autonomy and control the conditions of clinical practice, they resent and prevent outside qualified authorities from setting standards of medical care. This unfortunate situation would persist under a health-team model.

With the emergence of a Post-Physician Era a government panel of experts, drawn from the nation's most qualified medical researchers, could establish high standards of clinical care, program them into the computer, and thereby minimize the problem. Such a precedent already exists in that the Food and Drug Administration (FDA) currently determines which medications can be used by practitioners. Although one legitimately could disagree with the some of their decisions, most authorities recognize that the FDA has protected the public from many potentially harmful drugs. Under a medic-computer model in which the government would control the conditions of clinical work, high standards of care could be established to cover *all* types of medical practice. Furthermore, because an automated system of health care would collect all relevant clinical data, these government-appointed experts will possess more information to make more valid judgments than would their modern counterparts.

Because different hypotheses must be tested in clinical settings if medical knowledge is to expand, one might fear that if a single national panel of experts was the only group to set standards of care, medical progress would inevitably stagnate. This need not happen. Groups of experts with differing clinical perspectives could market government-sanctioned medical computer programs that could be purchased and utilized by local health care agencies. If researchers evaluated the effectiveness of each of these programs, medical progress would not be impeded. A medic-computer model could establish a compromise between our present situation in which physicians are relatively free to do what they please and a system of excessive uniformity.

Health Care Financing. From 1950 to 1973 the portion of our gross national product allocated to health care rose from 4.6 to 7.7 percent. During the same interval national medical expenditures increased from $12 to $94.1 billion per year (4). By 1980 this figure is expected to climb to as high as $200 billion and constitute 9.8 percent of the gross national product (9). It is no wonder that the escalating costs of providing medical services has generated public alarm. Numerous developments have been implicated for inflating health care expenditures, such as technological innovations, medical progress, higher wages, inflation, and increased consumer demands and expectations. However, many authorities believe that the present structure for delivering medical services fosters economic inefficiency (6, 8–14).

The reasons for this allegation are complex, and a thorough discussion of them is beyond the scope of this book. Nevertheless, several points are worth noting. Because physicians primarily control the operations and structure of our health care system, to a large extent they determine how medical expenditures will be allocated. Doctors have not exercised fiscal restraint for many reasons. In 1972 federal, state, and local governments paid 40.1 percent of all medical costs, while private insurance companies covered 24.8 percent of the bill (4). In the same year hospital care accounted for the largest portion or 38.9 percent of medical expenses (15). Nevertheless, the government has not provided doctors with sufficient incentives to reduce costs, nor have hospital administrators or insurance officials instituted rigorous economic controls (6). This situation is unlikely to change as long as physicians retain their authority over the health care system.

Because of the belief that the economic hardships experienced by most health care consumers can be resolved by simply channelling more funds into the medical service industry, individuals anticipate that national health insurance will alleviate the financial plight of American medicine. Unfortunately, the public debate over national health insurance has focused almost exclusively upon the scope of services to be covered, without seriously examining the fundamental organizational issues that have given rise to our fiscal dilemmas. Theoretically, the establishment of alternative financing mechanisms could provide an excellent opportunity to offer new cost-reducing incentives (6). I suspect, however, that these reforms will not materialize. Just as in the cases of Medicare and Medicaid, political realities will dictate that the ultimate form of national health insurance will accommodate significantly to the desires of the medical profession. Undoubtedly, given their power, doctors will still be able to insist that the program will not infringe greatly upon their economic and especially their medical autonomy. Government will be reluctant to control physicians' fees or to set limits on the types or quantities of tests and procedures that doctors would be allowed to execute. As a result, medical expenditures will continue to escalate. * I am not suggesting that government could not implement effective controls, but I think that they would be unlikely to do so as long as doctors maintain their hegemony over the health care system.

The economic impact of physician dominance also contributes to spiraling hospital bills. Inpatient costs are an important area to focus upon because they represent the largest segment of the nation's health care expenditures. In 1960 32.9 percent of all medical expenses went to providing hospital care; in 1973 this figure rose to 38.5 percent (4). Doctors who are trained largely in hospital settings find admitting patients more convenient and

---

* Because the outputs of the medical sector (e.g. improved health, alleviation of suffering) are difficult to quantify, it has been argued that cost-benefit analyses are of dubious value (4). Nevertheless, useful analyses have been executed (10, 14).

preferable than treating them on an ambulatory basis. Because health insurance usually favors inpatient coverage, strong incentives exist for doctors and patients to prefer inhospital care. Once patients are admitted, physicians demonstrate little regard for controlling expenditures (6); among other reasons, insurance companies or the government will frequently pay the bill. Even if the patient assumes the financial burden for his care, because of his dependency upon the physician and his lack of technical expertise, he is in no position to influence significantly the number of tests and procedures that will be performed. Consequently, doctors are not restrained by economic considerations.

Hospital administrators often are unable to control the physician's fiscal irresponsibility. Because 22 percent of beds are unoccupied (4), many administrators, especially those in community hospitals, are dependent upon physicians to admit patients and to utilize their facilities to the fullest to avert financial catastrophe. If administrators are to entice doctors to use their hospital, they must provide a wide range of expensive equipment and facilities. This results in many community hospitals duplicating costly medical services, even though many of these services are vastly underutilized. Because the economic survival of a hospital rests upon the good will of physicians, administrators are reluctant to impose fiscal limitations upon a medical staff, and therefore are relatively powerless to control the doctor's monetary abuses (6).

Placing the entire blame for escalating hospital and medical costs on doctors would be inaccurate and unfair. Many other reasons have led community hospital per diem costs to climb from $15.62 in 1950 to $105.21 in 1972 (4). For example, because hospitals increasingly possess record and conference rooms, laboratories, administrative offices, libraries, and computer facilities, proportionately less income-generating space is available. Seventy-five years ago 80 percent of a typical hospital's space was filled by patient beds; today this figure may be as low as 20 percent (9). Nevertheless, a physician-centered model has contributed largely to the fiscal crisis confronting American medicine. Because a Post-Physician Era would eliminate the medical profession's control of the health care system, planners in the future would be afforded innumerable opportunities to rectify many of our present economic dilemmas.

Bureaucracy. To most of us the term *bureaucracy* evokes images of lazy, rigid, faceless men whose primary task is to complicate the uncomplicated. Although "nobody" likes bureaucracies, we encourage their expansion whenever we want society to provide us with a greater number of goods or services. Throughout the world people increasingly expect government to underwrite the costs of medical care (16), and thus, bureaucracies continue to grow. Because the notion of bureaucracy has become so tainted we tend to overlook its *potential* merits. Worthwhile bureaucracies can facilitate higher standards of care and a more efficient use of human, institutional, and technical resources. At the same time, however, they can develop inflexible routines that do not allow themselves to deal efficiently with unusual situations. A fundamental dilemma confronting future medical administrators will be to establish bureaucracies that are strong enough to execute organizational procedures, yet fluid enough to respond helpfully to novel circumstances.

David Mechanic notes that the bureaucratic form most appropriate for the efficient organization of scientific medical practice is not the best form to deal with the supportive aspects of clinical work. He believes that most bureaucracies are structured to meet the requirements of the former, while only paying lip service to the needs of the latter. He maintains that administrative routines can and must be created that will satisfy patients' emotional, social, and educative health needs. What is most striking about Mechanic's analysis is that he tends to present the issue as an either-or proposition. He feels that when administrators set their *primary* objectives for a bureaucracy they must choose between technical and psychosocial goals (6).

I consider the first critical question to be if bureaucracies can be devised that will maximize *both* scientific and supportive medical functions. The second critical question is if health care bureaucracies have been designed primarily to meet the needs of consumers or providers of medical services. The answer to this question may offer us a clue as to why Mechanic conceptualizes the problem as one of choosing between scientific and supportive objectives. Because contemporary doctors have emphasized medicine's technical activities over its psychosocial functions, health care bureaucracies have reflected this bias. If a bureaucracy did not have to adjust excessively to the desires of the medical profession, it might become politically able to set the needs of patients as its major goal. Without physician dominance, a medic-computer model would allow administrators to create bureaucracies that effectively attend to both the technical and the supportive requirements of consumers.

Of course a medic-computer model will have its own bureaucratic dilemmas. One potential problem may be that the system will not be flexible enough to render decisions according to the unique characteristics of individual patients. For example, two patients may have nearly identical symptomatology, but one may be receptive to the idea of entering psychiatric treatment and the other may be insulted by the suggestion. If a medic conveyed a computer's recommendation of psychotherapy to this latter individual, he might induce the patient to flee altogether from the health care system. Although formal psychotherapy would have been the treatment of choice, emotional support from a medic would have been preferable to nothing. Unfortunately, the "insensitivity" of the computer's suggestion may have so alienated the patient that he would be unavailable to receive the medic's help. If medics automatically present patients with computer-generated recommendations without seriously considering their psychological impact, individualized care would be denied.

Another illustration of a bureaucratic danger under a medic-computer model would be if patient data are mistakenly programmed into the machine. Whether the patient gave an incorrect history to the computer* or the medic fed inaccurate information into the machine is irrelevant. Once the data are in

* Patients also give inaccurate histories to doctors (17).

the computer rectifying the error might be difficult. Subsequent automated medical decisions would be based upon inaccurate information, which in turn could have disastrous consequences. This problem may be minimized if the medic had the patient review a copy of his computerized history to detect any mistakes. This safeguard already has been utilized successfully at the University of Wisconsin Department of Psychiatry (18).

The two previous illustrations suggest that inflexibilities of the system would have to be monitored closely. Although bureaucrats, especially those who depend largely upon automation, tend to become irritated by any deviation from standardized routines, a health care bureaucracy could be created that places a high priority on adjusting to unique situations. In fact, devising such a bureaucracy may be one of the more challanging tasks of the New Medical Order. Despite the many bureaucratic problems that potentially could arise under a medic-computer model, this system would be free to correct these difficulties *without* having to cater to an excessively powerful interest group such as physicians. A medic-computer bureaucracy would be able to set the needs of consumers as its top priority.

Accessibility. A major deficiency of American medicine has been the relative inaccessibility of its health care services (6, 9–10, 19–20). The high costs of receiving medical care are frequently cited as an explanation for this problem (9). Per capita health expenditures have risen from $205.43 in 1967 to $339.56 in 1972. This figure is expected to reach $669.94 by 1980 (4). This suggests that for many individuals economic factors are a significant obstacle to obtaining medical services. Nevertheless, studies show that other factors influence utilization rates of medical services, such as their availability, the distance involved traveling to them, convenience of transportation, waiting times, the way patients are treated, and difficulty getting appointments (6).

An issue that deserves special attention is how patients initially enter a health care system. Formerly they contacted their family doctor; today many people have no one to whom they can turn.

In large measure this problem has arisen because specialization has all but replaced the general practitioner (19–20). In most circumstances physicians have chosen to specialize because they felt it was in their *own* rather than in society's best interest. Thus, because doctors primarily determine the conditions of medical practice, they have been able to get away with devising a health care system without any major regard for how patients could gain access to it.

In a Post-Physician Era the medic would serve as the patient's portal of entry into the health care system. Because of advances in communications technology that will most likely materialize by the 21st century, the patient would be able to establish contact with both a medic and a computer without having to leave his home. The absence of convenient transportation routes or a nearby clinic would not be a significant obstacle to those seeking medical attention. A medic-computer model would be more likely than a physician-centered model to function at full capacity around the clock. Machines are tireless and can operate 24 hours a day. Assuming that medics, like contemporary nurses, would have less control than physicians presently do over the health care system, they would have comparatively less autonomy over their schedules. Consequently, their hours, like those of hospital nurses, could be set primarily according to what patients need instead of what medics desire.

Accountability.   Assuming that ultimately practitioners should be accountable to those they serve, the organizational structure of any health care system must ensure adequate yet appropriate consumer controls. A brief examination of our current situation will reveal that these objectives are difficult to accomplish under a physician-centered model. Admittedly, patients do have some control over the actions of individual doctors, clinics, and hospitals; if they are dissatisfied, they can go elsewhere. Unfortunately, clients are not always in a position to know if they ought to be dissatisfied. Patients are able to evaluate some aspects of medical practice—namely, the physician's ability to meet their social, psychological, and educative health needs—but they lack the scientific expertise necessary to judge the doctor's technical skills. As a result, some patients unknowingly will remain with an incompetent physician simply because they are charmed by his bedside manner. Although patients are free to select the doctor of their choice, they are only semi-qualified to make that choice.

Given the inability of consumers to assess fully the competence of physicians, what societal mechanisms are available to hold doctors accountable for their actions? Theoretically, this responsibility rests with the judicial system and the medical profession. However, judges and juries are no better qualified to evaluate a physician's scientific abilities than are other laymen. Only doctors can adequately assess one another's technical skills. Unfortunately, the medical profession has been reluctant to assume this responsibility. Doctors' unwillingness to evaluate and, therefore, to criticize one another derives from several factors. If physicians fault their colleagues, they would invite retaliations from the accused, which in turn could lead to professional ostracism, decreased referrals, or providing dissatisfied patients with ammunition for potential malpractice suits. Physicians also recognize that all doctors, including themselves, inevitably commit errors. In detecting the apparent mistakes of others, the physician is inclined to feel, "There, but for the grace of God, go I" or "It might be my turn next." Furthermore, to evaluate adequately another physician's performance, direct observation is necessary. Not only does this consume a great deal of time, but more importantly, doctors find it infantilizing. After completing many years of arduous training a physician believes, "I'm a big boy now; I don't need to be watched." In summarizing doctors' attitudes, Freidson writes:

> Being supervised is synonymous with being a student. It implies not being trusted with one's responsibility. Indeed, to be granted freedom from supervision is a mark of being trusted, of being autonomous; in short, of being a professional. Being visible when the work itself requires it or where one himself so requests is acceptable, but anything more is uncomfortable, if not demeaning.

A professional does not lower himself by snooping into the affairs of colleagues and expects his colleagues to respect the privacy of his affairs (5, p. 180)

Finally, many doctors believe that professional unity is the best defense against public criticism, and therefore, to disrupt that unity will only generate more public criticism (5). Although doctors correctly believe they are the only ones qualified to judge the technical skills of other physicians, in practice it is unusual for them to do so. * Even when such intraprofessional monitoring does occur, it is rare for doctors to be fined, have their licenses taken away, or their hospital privileges revoked.

Opportunities for genuine and effective accountability may be enhanced under a medic-computer model. Because medics would conduct primarily supportive tasks and consumers are qualified to assess these tasks, patients legitimately could evaluate the medics' performance. If patients feel dissatisfied with a medic, they could go elsewhere. Simultaneously, researchers could appraise the effectiveness of a medical computer without having to worry about insulting its feelings.

Accountability applies not only to clinicians, but also to the bureaucracies in which they function. One of the major reasons for establishing effective accountability mechanisms is to increase the responsiveness of a health care system. As medical institutions become more complex they tend to become less responsive to patients' needs. One way to reduce this problem is by the use of ombudsmen. When patients have a complaint, they can communicate it to an ombudsman who in turn investigates the allegation and attempts to rectify it. Ombudsmen must be acquainted with the operations of a medical setting, its organizational structure, personnel, and available services. They also must be sensitive to the emotional and social needs of patients,

---

* Recently, physicians have been forced by the government to establish peer-monitoring groups called "Professional Standards Review Organizations". Although it is too early to know if these programs will materialize, I suspect that even if they do, the resistance of the medical profession will neutralize their potential effectiveness.

without harassing clinicians with unjust or trivial complaints (6). Although the reactions of physicians to ombudsmen vary widely, many doctors seem to resent their activities because they believe that they encroach upon their autonomy. Although the ombudsman concept has flourished in other fields (21), its use in medicine has been restricted to a few hospitals (22–23). Nevertheless, the ombudsman may play a greater role in medicine's future. With the increased growth of consumerism and as the public finds it progressively more difficult to contend with the complexities of obtaining health care, they not only may need, but actually demand, patient advocates. In addition, as doctors play a declining role in the delivery of medical services, physicians will exert less control over the health care system, and therefore, would be less able to prevent the utilization of ombudsmen.

Ombudsmen also could assist health planners by relaying frequently encountered consumer complaints to those in higher managerial positions. Administrators could then use this information to make personnel or structural changes that may alleviate reoccurring problems. Of course, accountability mechanisms may need to be established for ombudsmen themselves.

The ombudsmen concept is not the only way to improve the responsiveness of complex health bureaucracies. Another way the public can increase the responsiveness of a health care system is to participate in the management councils of hospitals, clinics, insurance companies, educational institutions, and so on. The thorny question of whether this should entail mere involvement or actual control is too complex to explore adequately in this book. Nevertheless, several principles ought to be considered. The relationship and distinction between responsibility, authority, and accountability must be kept in mind. If health care administrators are to be accountable to the public, the public must grant them the power to implement the program. Administrators cannot be held responsible unless they are given sufficient managerial authority. They must also be sufficiently knowledgeable to make appropriate decisions. Fundamental to the ability of consumers to set policies and of administrators to implement those policies is the need for accurate, reliable, valid, and available information.

Computers can assist both administrators and the public in the accumulation, analysis, and retrieval of such data. Furthermore, as the complexity of the health care system grows, automation will be increasingly necessary to provide relevant information. Although these principles are applicable to any form of health care delivery, they are especially well-suited to a medic-computer model because automation is central and essential to its operation.

Continuity of Care. One of the major deficiencies of our present medical system is the fragmented and uncoordinated nature of many clinical services (6, 10). Not only is inpatient and outpatient treatment conducted frequently by different practitioners, but at times these doctors do not even communicate with one another. With increasing specialization and group practice, many patients are without a specific physician who assumes overall responsibility for their care. Nevertheless, the medical profession still has the obligation to provide continuity of service.

Most authorities believe that difficult clinical tasks should be done by the people best trained to perform them. Under a physician-centered and especially a health-team model, the provision of scientific excellence and continuity of care are desirable, yet to some extent incompatible objectives. As David Mechanic explains, ". . .continuity of care is best assured when a small number of people provides care to a patient over time, but highest technical performance is achieved with a highly specialized division of labor and an elaborate referral system. Both values cannot be simultaneously optimized, and some decision must be made concerning their relative priorities" (6, p. 17).

Indeed, if one assumes that clinical skills can be delivered only by practitioners and that medical knowledge will continue to expand, the dilemma of having to choose between technical excellence and continuity of care will become an even greater issue in the future. A medic-computer model, however, may extricate us from this problem. Because the machine will offer the highest quality of available medical decision making, while being able to synthesize clinical data, * the continuity of scientific care will be assured. Because patients will affiliate with a specific medic, the latter will be able to provide continuity of supportive care. As a result, the dilemma posed by Mechanic could be over come by a machine-medic symbiosis; a Post-Physician Era could offer technical excellence without sacrificing continuity of care.

EVOLVING PATTERNS OF HEALTH CARE. In planning for a future medical care system we must not only consider general organizational issues, but also anticipate the evolving health needs of the populace. Future health care policies should be made with an awareness of changing patterns of illness as well as the availability of new treatment methods. Although these topics are too extensive to discuss comprehensively in this book, several relevant issues may be worth examining to illustrate some of the important problems we should consider in planning for the New Medical Order.

Changing Patterns of Illness. In 1900 the leading causes of death in the United States were influenza and pneumonia, tuberculosis, gastroenteritis, and heart disease (24). Seventy-two years later they were heart disease, cancer, stroke, and accidents (4). The change in the "top four" reflects a number of factors. The discovery of antibiotics has lowered the mortality rate due to pneumonia and tuberculosis. Advances in nutrition, housing, and sanitation have decreased the seriousness of these diseases, as well as influenza and gastroenteritis. Partially because of these developments, the average life span of the populace has increased from 47.3 years in 1900 to 71.2 years in 1972 (4). As a result, disorders of older age, such as cancer, stroke, and heart disease, have become more prevalent. Technological changes, which have

---

* Later in this chapter this issue will be examined more extensively when medical computer data banks are discussed.

very little direct relationship to medicine, have contributed to the rise of accidents and to some forms of cancer.

Over the next 50 years the prevalence of the "top four" illnesses will continue to change. Although the exact nature of these variations is unpredictable, undoubtedly biomedical discoveries, as well as social and technological changes, will influence future disease patterns. Recent advances in immunology, virology, and chemotherapy may lead to a cure for many types of cancer. A deeper understanding of the neurological and biochemical basis of major psychiatric syndromes, such as schizophrenia and mood disorders, may help to decrease the severity of these illnesses. Many conditions affecting the central nervous system, such as Parkinson's disease and multiple sclerosis, may be cured by medication. Genetic discoveries and improved prenatal care may reduce significantly the infant mortality rate.

As medical advances prolong life, chronic ailments will become a greater concern to those who deliver health care services. Greater attention may be focused upon emphysema arthritic disorders, aging, and antisocial behavior. The increasing mobility of the populace and the breakdown of communal and family ties will deprive individuals of stable traditions, mores, and values. These developments may diminish those neurotic disorders in which a rigid cultural ethic and repression allegedly play major etiological roles. The fluidity, flux, and change that will characterize future societies (2) may lead to an increase of those neurotic disturbances in which cultural instability supposedly is a significant causative factor. We also may witness the "internationalization of disease" as global travel becomes more pervasive; illnesses once thought to exist only in remote areas of the world may find their way into the United States. And finally, one cannot help but wonder if expanded space travel will introduce a wide variety of previously unknown ailments.

Contrary to what some have predicted (25), we will witness changing patterns of illness, rather than the elimination of disease. Although mortality rates due to infections have been on the decline, to extrapolate this trend and to conclude that inevitably infectious diseases and the pathogens that cause them will be eradicated would be a mistake (26–27). Because older people are more susceptible to infections and the longevity of the populace will continue to rise, infectious diseases may become a growing, rather than a declining, problem. Although antibiotics are useful in eradicating pathogenic agents, many bacteria are becoming drug resistant. Unfortunately, antibiotics give the illusion of controlling infectious diseases. As a result, for example people often abstain from taking safety precautions against gonorrhea on the false expectation that penicillin could readily cure the illness. Consequently, the prevalence of gonorrhea continues to escalate (28–29). Even if we could eradicate some pathogenic bacteria, nonpathogens can be transformed into or replaced by even more dangerous ones for which an effective treatment might not be available. Thus, future therapeutic objectives should be aimed toward the control, rather than the elimination of infectious diseases. As Koprowski has observed, "Man has to live with his infections in a state of ecological bliss" (27).

Changing Patterns of Treatment.   As the patterns of disease will be modified by medical, social, and technological change, so too will the patterns of treatment used to cure them. Medical care can be divided into four stages. Stage one is the prevention of disease, accidents, stress, and other causes of illness. Stage two is the early treatment of diseases before they become serious enough to require hospitalization. Stage three refers to acute care of severe illness that usually necessitates hospitalization. Stage four includes postacute, convalescent, rehabilitative, and terminal care. These services are delivered in a variety of settings, such as nursing and convalescent homes, chronic disease hospitals, and rehabilitation centers. Although a detailed discussion of these four stages can be found elsewhere (10), a few thoughts about them may be relevant to the future of medicine.

The implementation of preventive health programs (Stage one) requires a centralized coordinated effort, which cannot be accomplished as long as private physicians, who work in isolation, dominate the health care system. With the decline of the solo practitioner (30) and as the responsibility for medical care shifts from the private to the public sector (31), the opportunity to execute preventive health programs will be enhanced. The utilization of computers on a widespread basis will facilitate the collection of epidemiological data that in turn will augment the effectiveness of preventive health measures (32).

Although future developments may increase the opportunities to execute preventive health activities and although at first glance these programs sound appealing, we should be cautious about implementing them. When considering the many different types of preventive health programs, we must distinguish between those of potential merit and those of dubious value. For instance, the indiscriminate use of periodic health examinations may create as many problems as they solve. The assumptions that these examinations diminish the possibility of serious illnesses developing and ultimately reduce the costs of providing medical care have yet to be validated (33–34). In addition, there is little value in screening for a disease for which effective treatment is either unavailable or nonexistent. (At present there is minimal evidence that the early detection of asymptomatic diabetes will allow the physician to alter the ultimate course of the disorder [24, 33–34].) At least for some people, discovering that one has a disease, especially an untreatable disease, may have a devastating effect. The transition from person to patient may encourage the individual to assume the role of an invalid, even though one's actual physical state remains the same. This latter consideration becomes especially important if one realizes that inevitable diagnostic errors can lead to "false positive" results. Thus, an individual could become overwrought about a disease he does not even have (34). For a society to provide screening procedures that detect an illness and not have the resources available to treat it borders on immorality (24, 33). Of course, some preventive health measures are potentially valuable, but they must be selectively and judiciously executed.

The early treatment of disease (Stage two) may play an even greater role in medicine's future. From 1962 to 1972 outpatient visits rose by 121 percent (4, 15), and several developments may accelerate this trend. New pharmacological discoveries may allow a greater number of patients to be treated on an ambulatory basis. If the quantity of hospital beds continues to decline (4), doctors may be forced to see more people as outpatients (6). In the more distant future advances in communication and computer technology may permit patients to be treated at home who formerly would have required hospitalization. Finally—although I cannot give any evidence to support this contention—I suspect that the most important variable is that we are becoming a more health conscious society. If so, even more people will seek Stage two clinical services.

Although most authorities believe that encouraging patients to obtain early treatment is warranted both medically and economically (10), others are less convinced (6). Whether early treatment is justified is a vital question, because important policy decisions rest upon the answer. If early treatment is useful, future health care planners should allocate a greater portion of fiscal, technological, and professional resources to these endeavors. But if the value of early treatment has been overestimated, alternative priorities should prevail. Although there are no definitive conclusions to this controversy, the issue is so relevant to medicine's future, briefly examining both sides of this debate is worthwhile.

Advocates of early treatment can show that many patients are spared a great deal of suffering by obtaining prompt medical attention. For example, the early treatment of syphilis can prevent the subsequent occurrence of more serious cardio-vascular and neurological complications (35). Similarly, many experts believe that by receiving intensive psychiatric care, distressed individuals can avoid developing more severe emotional difficulties (36). Pessimists maintain that the ultimate course of many illnesses, such as hypertension, diabetes, and schizophrenia, are unaffected by early therapeutic interventions. To a large extent both the proponents and the opponents of early treatment are correct. Its advantages vary according to the particular disease under consideration. Some illnesses are helped by early treatment; others are not. Another issue to be weighed is whether the effectiveness of early treatment is measured in terms of short-term gains or long-range accomplishments. For example, proper insulin therapy may prevent many diabetics from going into coma, but it probably does not alter the ultimate course of their disease. When evaluating the medical utility of early treatment, one has to consider not only the specific illnesses involved, but also the criteria upon which the assessment are made.

The basic argument about the economic value of early treatment is whether the provision of extensive Stage-two care reduces the need for costly hospitalization. Advocates of early treatment note that the introduction of comprehensive outpatient services at Columbia Point in Boston decreased hospital admissions by 69 percent and hospital bed days by 80 percent. Patients in Kaiser-Permanente's prepaid ambulatory care program spent half the time in the hospital that nonparticipants did (10). These lower admission and bed occupancy rates are estimated to account for a 15 to 20 percent reduction of costs when compared to a similar socioeconomic group receiving more traditional medical services (6). Although these savings accrue from the decreased use of hospitalization, one cannot be sure that the provision of early treatment is the principal reason for this reduction. Skeptics point out that Kaiser has a lower bed-patient ratio than do more traditional practices. The relative scarcity of beds undoubtedly forces doctors to admit patients less frequently and to discharge them more rapidly. Furthermore, if early treatment reduces the need for hospitalization, one would expect higher ambulatory utilization rates among Kaiser participants. Although available data does not allow for an exact comparison, outpatient utilization rates among Kaiser patients are equal to, if not slightly lower than, those who receive typical medical services. At both Kaiser and Columbia Point considerable group pressure exists that encourages physicians to avoid admitting their patients (6). Thus, it is questionable if the savings derived from decreased hospital utilization could result either from the existence of comprehensive early treatment programs or from other significant variables. Before any firm conclusions can be drawn the medical and economic benefits of early treatment should be more carefully investigated.

Finally, we must consider if the emphasis placed on avoiding acute hospitalization (Stage three) is always in the patient's best interests. Although nobody would justify needless admissions, if systematic pressure is exerted upon clinicians to abstain from hospitalizing patients, some consumers will be denied the potential benefits that only inpatient care can offer (6, 37). The types of medical procedures that are best accomplished on an ambulatory basis must be distinguished from those optimally performed within a hospital. As this knowledge accumulates, hospitals may contain a greater number of specialty services. Already we have seen that cardiac care, intensive care, renal dialysis, trauma, and rehabilitation units are becoming more prevalent in many facilities (38).

For patients who must be hospitalized, boredom is a significant problem; except for a short visit by a physician and a brief injection by a nurse, patients spend most of their days languishing in a bed with very little to do. Patients could use this wasted time to participate on a voluntary basis in a wide range of health related educational and psychological programs. Lectures and discussion groups could be established for patients who suffer from similar disorders. They could be taught about their illnesses and learn how others have coped with them. While conducting these programs, physicians, nurses, or medics could acquire a deeper understanding of their patients and some of the practical problems they face in contending with their diseases. Group therapy already has been utilized successfully with medically hospitalized children to relieve anxiety, detect psychological problems, and diminish feelings of loneliness that often accompany hospitalization (39). Because the hospital is a temporary total environment for patients (37), we can maximize not only its medical, but also its educational and psychological potential.

According to the 1968 report of the National Advisory Council on Health Facilities a high proportion of Stage-four treatment (i.e., postacute, convalescent, rehabilitative, and terminal care) presently conducted in acute general hospitals could be provided equally well and at less expense by long-term facilities and home care programs (10). As the life span of the populace and the prevalence of chronic diseases increase, the demand for these institutions and programs may be greater than ever before. To function optimally they ought to have ready access to the services offered by acute general hospitals. Currently, this usually necessitates that Stage-four treatment facilities be in close *geographic* proximity to institutions that offer sophisticated care. In the future, however, developments in telecommunications may alter this requirement so that *electronic* proximity will suffice. Furthermore, because Stage-four treatment is frequently inadequate, improving these facilities should be an important goal for the New Medical Order.

NATIONAL MEDICAL DATA BANK. Methods by which medical records are stored and retrieved will change. The increased mobility of the citizenry, the possibility of even greater compartmentalization of clinical services, the advent of national health insurance, the potential for enhancing biomedical research, and the growing use of computers may lead to the establishment of a national medical data bank (NMDB). The potential benefits and dangers of a central file are so great to patients—as well as to society—that this topic deserves special consideration.

An automated national medical data bank would store all of the patient's medical records so that authorized personnel could rapidly obtain accurate, legible, and relevant clinical information. With the patient's written consent, this data could be transmitted from a central computer to a display-printer terminal situated in the office of his physician, medic, or other health care professional. The local practitioner also could send new clinical information to the NMDB to update the patient's central record. The patient or his legal representative (in the case of minors or incompetents) could decide *voluntarily* to have their records stored in the NMDB. Each participant could be identified by his social security number and the first four letters of his last name.* Similarly, all

---

* This system is used by the Internal Revenue Service in processing tax returns.

practitioners in the country would register their social security
and medical license numbers to be allowed to acquire or add information to the patient's file. Special plastic identification cards for
both the health care professional and the patient could be inserted
simultaneously into the local terminal to receive the patient's
medical record (40).

The advantages of a computerized national medical data bank
are numerous. An automated method could rectify the deficiencies of our current system, in which medical records often are
illegible, inaccurate, incomplete, and inaccessible (41). The rapid
availability of the patient's clinical file would greatly facilitate the
provision of emergency care, whether the practitioner was or was
not familiar with the case. As the mobility of the populace
increases, more patients will receive treatment from health care
professionals unacquainted with their medical history. An NMDB
will help to overcome this problem and assist in identifying
patients who have been given a drug or treatment subsequently
found to be harmful, possess an illness for which a new treatment
has been discovered, and have a particularly rare blood type for
which a transfusion could be donated. And finally, a national
medical data bank would facilitate clinical and epidemiological
research (40).

Despite the many advantages of an NMDB, the centralization
and computerization of clinical information may threaten the
patient's right to privacy.* Although the advent of an NMDB
will raise many new and very justifiable concerns about the future
confidentiality of medical records, these fears may be exaggerated.
In a comprehensive study computers were found to have caused
much less erosion of privacy than is commonly believed (42).
Moreover, we should recognize that patient privacy using non-
automated records is being widely infringed upon already (40,
43, 46–52). Insurance companies can see the entire medical file
of any of their clients. A little known organization, the Medical

---

* In this book the right to privacy will refer to the patient's claim that he is
entitled to decide when, what, and to whom his medical and psychological
records may be communicated.

Information Bureau, provides more than 700 insurance companies with clinical data and information about the financial affairs and personal pursuits of some 12 million Americans. It is nearly impossible for citizens to find out what information about themselves is possessed and transmitted by this organization (44.–46). Although the Medical Information Bureau provides data to insurance companies only, anybody, who for whatever nefarious reasons wants to view a patient's medical record, can do so. A patient's chart can be stolen or obtained by bribing a physician, nurse, or secretary. At one time it would have seemed farfetched to believe that the government would steal medical records; history has taught us otherwise. Government violations of patient confidentiality are not limited to Watergate-like episodes. Although the Fourth Amendment prohibits arbitrary government intrusions into our private affairs, the government subpoenas medical records, inspects them for Medicare and Medicaid payments and examines them as part of utilization review procedures.

The establishment of an NMDB and the threats to privacy that may accompany this development may arise in the very near future. The enactment of national health insurance will probably lead to the creation of an NMDB, which then may be tied to computers administering social welfare agencies and possibly even the Internal Revenue Service (50). Increasing centralized automated information collection will create new opportunities for transgressing our already diminishing privacy. Given this predicament, there are four basic available options. First, we can legally forbid the creation of an NMDB. However, because of the numerous advantages of such a bank, I would be against this approach. Second, we can establish an NMDB without much concern for potential infringements of confidentiality. This alternative is equally undesirable. Third, an NMDB would be developed, but *only* if the confidentiality of medical records would be *completely* guaranteed. Although this policy may seem to be the best to pursue, because no absolute guarantees could ever be provided, in practice it would preclude the establishment of an NMDB. A fourth, and in my estimation the most favorable approach, would be to create an NMDB that substantially protects the individual's right to privacy.

If an NMDB is to be relatively safe from abuse, some precautions must be implemented. Because clinical information would be more accessible, special efforts will be required to ensure that a patient's computerized file will be accurate, possess only relevant information, and be frequently updated. To improve the reliability of automated records and to give consumers some control over the information being circulated about them, individuals should have access to their own dossiers and be allowed to challenge their accuracy (46, 50–53). This principle has been recognized in the Federal Fair Credit Reporting Act, which has reduced some of the abuses that have resulted from the indiscriminate transmission of personal information by consumer-reporting companies (49). Data in a patient's file should be reviewed systematically and periodically to purge distorted, inaccurate, irrelevant, or archaic material (47, 49). This becomes especially important for psychological data. School records that are filled with subjective judgments could plague an individual throughout his life. A withdrawn child, who may have been examined for a possible diagnosis of childhood schizophrenia, may grow up to be normal. However, that tentative diagnosis made at an early age could damage his reputation 30 years later when he seeks political office (52). A national panel on medical records, consisting of laymen, attorneys, and health care professionals, could determine what information would be helpful and legitimate to include within a patient's file. This committee also could establish guidelines for the appropriate dissemination of clinical information (52). Computerized medical data may need to be divided into differential levels of confidentiality (40, 47, 54). Highly sensitive data should be available only to those directly responsible for treating the patient. Moreover, clinicians should obtain only information they are able to understand by virtue of their training and experience. For example, psychological test data can be misinterpreted and thereby abused by doctors, paraprofessionals, or medics who do not fully comprehend the meaning of this material (47). However, less sensitive data, such as nutritional and housing information, may be deemed useful and legitimate for selected government agencies. But anonymity must prevail when transmitting this data as well as medical information to clinical researchers.

In addition to establishing certain policy guidelines, technological safeguards will have to be employed to minimize unauthorized intrusions into a patient's automated medical record. Several protective features have been suggested. There is some evidence that computers radiate when in operation, and that by using eavesdropping techniques these emanations can be captured and subsequently deciphered. This danger can be overcome either by shielding the central processor and local terminals with metallic paper or by utilizing circuit suppressors and filters. The use of scrambling devices and codes may protect information that is transmitted via communication wires. If these precautions are to be employed, the number of individuals cognizant of the cryptographic system will have to be limited. Legitimate entry privileges into the data bank will have to be monitored. Practitioners could be required to identify themselves by using a special terminal code number or by having their finger or voice prints scanned. Closed circuit television also could be used to observe those who request information. A "buddy system" could be established whereby two health care professionals are needed to gain access to confidential medical data. Furthermore, two keys could be utilized in a manner resembling the procedure currently used in unlocking safety deposit boxes. All inquiries into a patient's central file could be logged by a computer and entered into a record to have a permanent register that could be inspected in case suspicion arises over the inappropriate use of the data bank. Although many of these protective features already are available (47, 54–55), profitminded companies may be reluctant to install them unless they are required to do so by law (43). The utilization of these technical devices must be considered before the accurate costs of establishing an NMDB can be determined (40).

Some authors believe that the right to privacy is so vital that most of these steps must be taken before national, regional, or hospital medical data banks are established (47, 56). However, to implement even some of these legal and technological measures becomes an incredibly complex and expensive task. Consequently, to insist upon the provision of *all* of these procedures as a prerequisite for the creation of automated data banks would essentially preclude the possibility of collecting, maintaining, and transmitting computerized medical records.* More important, we should not perpetuate the illusion that a system, whether automated or manual, can ever be designed that will guarantee both absolute confidentiality *and* high quality medical care. Regardless of the prevailing health care model there always will be numerous people (e.g., physicians, nurses, medics) who will have a legitimate reason to view a patient's medical record. If too many obstacles to obtaining clinical information are erected, patient care inevitably will suffer. The establishment of excessive barriers to information may deter or even prevent many health care professionals from acquiring data that are absolutely necessary for them to possess if they are to deliver decent medical services. The patient's legitimate right to privacy must be measured against the patient's equally legitimate right to excellent health care (53). Although reasonable steps must be taken to maximize the confidentiality of clinical information, the zealous insistence upon absolute guarantees will have deleterious consequences. What good would it be if we established a rigid and elaborate system wherein a patient's privacy is so sacrosanct that he dies with his civil rights intact?

I also share Dr. Lawrence Weed's concern that our society needs to adopt a fresh attitude toward the notion of privacy (53). As the citizenry becomes increasingly aware that their rights to medical confidentiality are being infringed upon and that automated clinical services may provide new opportunities for these rights to be violated, people may become more reluctant to divulge sensitive but vital medical information to health professionals. Without this data, practitioners will be unable to provide high quality clinical care. I concur with Dr. Weed's suggestion that we

---

* It also would present a formidable obstacle to the creation of a medic-computer model.

foster an ethos of openness rather than secrecy about personal medical information.

I am not suggesting that we violate people's legal rights to confidentiality; the Fourth Amendment protects these rights, and we should continue to protect them. I am proposing that patients be taught that hiding personal clinical information can be harmful to themselves, to their relatives, and to society. The unwillingness of many people to discuss the existence of a mentally ill family member tends to alienate the patient from himself and his community and place an unnecessary emotional burden upon the patient, his relatives, and friends (57). A study of psychiatric inpatients revealed that discussing their difficulties openly, honestly, and freely among themselves decreased their feelings of being "the only ones in the world with these problems" and, therefore, seemed to accelerate their recoveries (58). President and Mrs. Ford did their country a great service by publicly disclosing her breast cancer and mastectomy. The sense of shame traditionally associated with this condition was diminished, and many women were encouraged to have their own breasts examined. Because early detection of breast cancer can save lives, undoubtedly many people are living today who otherwise would have died. By openly discussing the issue, President Ford set an excellent example for other men—namely, that males should not be ashamed of women who have had a breast removed. Open discussion of medical or psychiatric problems enhances the patient's and the public's willingness to accept and be tolerant of disease and, more importantly, to do something constructive about it. Although medical professionals should make every effort to protect their patient's *legal* rights to privacy, they also should exercise their *moral* obligation to encourage their patients to be open and honest in talking about their illnesses. Indeed, Philip Slater may be right when he observed, "We seek more and more privacy, and feel more and more alienated when we get it" (59, p. 7).

SUMMARY. Although the greater use of medical technology and allied health personnel will generate new problems, it also will afford us fresh and previously unavailable opportunities to reform the organizational structure of our health care system. Changing patterns of disease and treatment will affect the delivery of medical services.

Whether man will respond constructively and effectively to these developments may determine if the New Medical Order will be a humane alternative future. To a large extent our capacity to accomplish this objective may depend not only upon our willingness to anticipate and plan for the future, but also upon our ability to adapt psychologically to a rapidly changing society. As Eric Hoffer has written, "We can never be really prepared for that which is wholly new. We have to adjust ourselves, and every radical adjustment is a crisis in self-esteem. . . .It needs inordinate self-confidence to face drastic change without inner trembling" (60, p. 9). Whether we have this strength may determine the degree to which we create a health care utopia or a medical dystopia.

NOTES

1. Erikson, E. H. (1968). *Identity: Youth and Crisis.* New York: Norton.

2. Toffler, A. (1971). *Future Shock.* New York: Bantam.

3. Roszak, T. (1968). *The Making of the Counter Culture: Reflections on the Technocratic Society and Its Youthful Opposition.* Garden City, N. J.: Doubleday.

4. Eisenberg, B. S., and P. Aherne (eds.) (1974). *Socioeconomic Issues of Health '74.* Chicago: American Medical Association.

5. Freidson, E. (1972). *Profession of Medicine: A Study of the Sociology of Applied Knowledge.* New York: Dodd, Mead.

6. Mechanic, D. (1972). *Public Expectations and Health Care: Essays on the Changing Organization of Health Services.* New York: Wiley-Interscience.

7. Fuchs, V. R. (1968). "The Growing Demand for Medical Care." *New England Journal of Medicine,* 279:190–195.

8. Sedgwick, P. (1974). "Medical Individualism." *The Hastings Center Studies,* 2(3):69–80.

9. Ribicoff, A., and P. Danaceau (1973). *The American Medical Machine*. New York: Harrow.

10. Chase, A. (1971). *The Biological Imperatives: Health, Politics, and Human Survival*. Baltimore: Penguin.

11. Greenberg, S. (1971). *The Quality of Mercy: A Report on the Critical Condition of Hospital and Medical Care in America*. New York: Atheneum.

12. Kennedy, E. M. (1972). *In Critical Condition: The Crisis in America's Health Care*. New York: Simon and Schuster.

13. Tunley, R. (1966). *The American Health Scandal*. New York: Harper & Row.

14. Anderson, O. W. (1972). *Health Care: Can There Be Equity?* New York: Wiley-Interscience.

15. Alevizos, G., R. J. Walsh, and P. Aherne (eds.) (1973). *Socioeconomic Issues of Health*. Chicago: American Medical Association.

16. Mechanic, D. (1974). *Politics, Medicine, and Social Science*. New York: Wiley-Interscience.

17. Gottlieb, G. L., R. F. Beers, Jr., C. Bernecker, and M. Samter (1972). "An Approach to Automation of Medical Interviews." *Computers and Biomedical Research*, 5:99–107.

18. Greist, J. H., L. J. Van Cura, and N. P. Kneppreth (1973). "A Computer Interview for Emergency Room Patients." *Computers and Biomedical Research*, 6:257–265.

19. Field, M. G. (1971). "The Health Care System of Industrial Society: The Disappearance of the General Practitioner and Some Implications." In E. Mendelsohn, J. P. Swazey, and I. Taviss (eds.), *Human Aspects of Biomedical Innovation*. Cambridge: Harvard University Press. Pp. 156–180.

20. Stead, E. A., Jr. (1973). "Family Practice: One View." In J. Graves (ed.), *The Future of Medical Education*. Durham, N.C.: Duke University Press. Pp. 143–154.

21. Kaufman, M. T. (1974). "The Two Kinds of Ombudsman—One Is Tough." *New York Times*, November 17. Section E, p. 12.

22. *Hospital Tribune* (1973). "Complaints in Hospital? Dial C-A-R-E on Hotline," 7(13):24.

23. *American Medical News* (1973). "Medicine's Week: Montreal Jewish Hospital," 16(45):2.

24. Sidel, V. W. (1971). "New Technologies and the Practice of Medicine." In E. Mendelsohn, J. P. Swazey, and I. Taviss (eds.), *Human Aspects of Biomedical Innovation*. Cambridge: Harvard University Press. Pp. 131–155.

25. Bellamy, E. (1926). *Looking Backward 2000–1887*. Boston: Houghton Mifflin.

26. Saliba, N. A., and W. H. Anderson (1970). "The Future Care of Tuberculosis Patients." *Journal of the American Medical Association*, 214:354–357.

27. Koprowski, H. (1963). "Future of Infectious and Malignant Diseases." In E. W. Gordon (ed.), *Man and His Future*. Boston: Little, Brown. Pp. 196–216.

28. Lucas, J. B. (1972). "The National Venereal Disease Problem." *Medical Clinics of North America*, **56**:1073–1086.

29. Barrett-Connor, E. (1974). "The Epidemiology and Control of Gonorrhea and Syphilis: A Reappraisal." *Preventive Medicine*, **3**:102–121.

30. Ehrlich, G. E. (1973). "Health Challenges of the Future." *The Annals of the American Academy of Political and Social Science*, **408**:70–82.

31. Harvard University Program on Technology and Society (1968). *Implications of Biomedical Technology, Research Review Number 1*. Cambridge (mimeograph).

32. Collen, M. F. (1969). "Development of Health Systems-II." In J. F. Dickson III, and J. H. U. Brown (eds.), *Future Goals of Engineering in Biology and Medicine*. New York: Academic. Pp. 279–285.

33. Thorner, R. M. (1969). "Whither Multiphasic Screening?" *New England Journal of Medicine*, **280**:1037–1042.

34. White, D. (1968). "Twenty Years After or Cloud Nine Attained." In G. McLachlan, and R. A. Shegog (eds.), *Computers in the Service of Medicine, Volume II*. London: Oxford University Press. Pp. 185–194.

35. Heyman, A. (1966). "Spirochetal Diseases." In T. R. Harrison, R. D. Adams, I. L. Bennett, Jr., W. H. Resnick, G. W. Thorn, and M. M. Wintrobe (eds.), *Principles of Internal Medicine*. New York: McGraw-Hill. Pp. 1628–1641.

36. Caplan, G. (1964). *Principles of Preventive Psychiatry*. New York: Basic Books.

37. Maxmen, J. S., G. J. Tucker, and M. D. LeBow (1974). *Rational Hospital Psychiatry: The Reactive Environment*. New York: Brunner/Mazel.

38. Weil, M. H., H. Shubin, and D. Stewart (1969). "Patient Monitoring and Intensive Care Units-I." In J. F. Dickson III, and J. H. U. Brown (eds.), *Future Goals of Engineering in Biology and Medicine*. New York: Academic. Pp. 232–246.

39. *Medical World News* (1973). "Group Therapy Eases Pediatric Stay," **14**(18): 55–56.

40. Freed, R. N. (1969). "A Legal Structure for A National Medical Data Center." *Boston University Law Review*, **49**:79–94.

41. Weed, L. L. (1969). *Medical Records, Medical Education, and Patient Care*. Cleveland: Press of Case Western Reserve University.

42. Westin, A. F., and M. A. Baker (1972). *Databanks in A Free Society*. New York: Quadrangle.

43. Greenwalt, K. (1974). "Privacy and Its Legal Protections." *The Hastings Center Studies*, **2**(3):45–68.

44. Pascoe, J. (1974). "MIB: It Has 12 Million Americans at Its Fingertips." *Prism*, **2**(6):28–33, 48, 51.

45. Entmacher, P. S. (1973). "Computerized Insurance Records: The Duty to Withhold." *Hastings Center Report*, **3**(5):8–9.

46. Gutman, J. S. (1973). "Computerized Insurance Records: The Right to Know." *Hastings Center Report*, 3(5):9–10.

47. Miller, A. R. (1971). *The Assault on Privacy: Computers, Data Banks, and Dossiers*. New York: New American Library.

48. Lyons, R. D. (1973). "Medical Records: They May Be Bad for You." *New York Times*, October 7. Section E, p. 3.

49. Ervin, S. J. (1974). "Civilized Man's Most Valued Right." *Prism*, 2(6): 14–17, 34.

50. Miller, A. R. (1974). "A Nation of Datamaniacs." *Prism*, 2(6):18–21, 56–59.

51. Jackson, C. B. (1974). "Guardians of Medical Data." *Prism*, 2(6):38–44.

52. Freedman, A. M. (1974). "Of Special Concern to Psychiatry. . . ." *Prism*, 2(6):35–37.

53. Weed, L. L. (1974). "The Public's Needs *Must* Be Met." *Prism*, 2(6): 22–26.

54. *Computers and Medicine* (1974). " 'Vital'—A Real Time Hospital Information System," 3(4):1–2.

55. *Massachusetts Physician* (1972). "Computer Privacy," 31(10):28.

56. Rumsey, J. M. (1974). "The Patient's Trust *Must* Be Protected." *Prism*, 2(6):22–26.

57. Bachman, B. (1971). "Re-Entering the Community: A Former Patient's View." *Hospital and Community Psychiatry*, 22:35–38.

58. Maxmen, J. S. (1973). "Group Therapy as Viewed by Hospitalized Patients." *Archives of General Psychiatry*, 28:404–408.

59. Slater, P. (1970). *The Pursuit of Loneliness*. Boston: Beacon.

60. *Kaiser Aluminum News* (1966). "The Anatomy of Change," 24(1):7–9.

4

THE ELECTRONIC
HOUSE CALL————————————

Future historians may record the latter third of the 20th century as a period in which communication technology revolutionized health care delivery. If this radical transformation is to materialize, however, an infinite array of unforeseeable events must occur. Yet even if communication technology fails to revolutionize the provision of clinical services, it will have a significant impact upon medicine's future.

MEDICAL COMMUNICATIONS TODAY.   On July 5, 1967 a patient in France received an electrocardiogram. This seemingly unspectacular event would have escaped notice except for the fact that the EKG was transmitted via communications satellite to Washington D.C., where it was analyzed by a computer and the results were returned to France. All of this occured within 30 seconds. (1) A year later a computer at New York's Mount Sinai Medical Center interpreted the EKGs of patients who lived in a small West Virginia community. Conventional telephone lines electronically transmitted the electrocardiogram. This program was highly successful; within two minutes West Virginia general practitioners received expert EKG readings. Previously they had to rely upon the mails for a cardiologist's interpretations, which took approximately two weeks. The cost for a routine hospital EKG was approximately $25; with this computer-communication linkup the price was reduced to $10 per reading (2).

Both of these experiments were significant because they demonstrated the contributions that advanced communication technology could play in the delivery of future health care services. They also showed that the integration of computer and communication technology allows for the transmission of highly technical information across wide geographic areas. To acquire an expert consultation physicians and other health care professionals no longer have to be in the same community; they can be located on opposite ends of the globe.

The linkage of computer and communication technology has not been limited to the interpretation of electrocardiograms. At the National Institute of Health a program has been devised in which physicians acquire up-to-date information on medication compatibility, drug identification, pediatric burn therapy, and medical diagnosis. Using a push button telephone as a computer terminal, the physician dials a central time-sharing computer. The machine asks a series of questions by means of a voice recording, which the doctor hears over his telephone receiver. By pushing certain buttons or by using dialer cards, the physician feeds the appropriate questions or data back into the central computer, which then returns the desired information (3–5). This program, known as an audio-response or a voice-answerback system, allows small medical facilities and even individual practitioners who cannot afford to rent or purchase a computer on their own to have access to the machine at a reasonable cost. They do not have to contend with complicated operating procedures, machine unavailability, or lack of technical experts. The telephone, when integrated with a time-sharing computer, provides health care personnel with the services of the machine without the responsibility of having to maintain it. (5)

A telephone's versatility can be expanded by combining it with a camera, cathode ray tube, and a video processing unit to yield a picturephone. Phonovision, or videophone, as it also has been called, allows people to see as well as to hear one another. It has been used successfully in several medical centers, enabling parents to visit their hospitalized children electronically and permitting physicians to transmit visual images of EKGs, X-rays, patient charts, and so on (6).

The most extensive use of videophones has been by urologist Irving Bush at Chicago's Cook County Hospital. Ten picturephone stations are located throughout the facility, including the emergency and recovery rooms, a cystoscopy suite, a patient ward, and in Dr. Bush's office. Without having to leave his office, he is able to keep abreast of activities within his department that are occurring in widely diverse places. In the first six months of operation the system has been well received by medical staff and patients alike. Physicians have not had to race to distant parts of the hospital to handle an emergency. Instead they use their videophone. In a sense they can be in two places at once.

Phonovision can transmit X-rays that are remarkably sharp and easy to interpret. When nurses are in short supply or unavailable because of an emergency, picturephones also can be utilized to monitor individual patients or even an entire ward (7-8).

What has been most gratifying about this phonovision system is that patients have not felt that it leads to the further dehumanization of medical care. Instead, they believe it has enhanced their relationship to the physician. As Bush has pointed out, many doctors who visit hospitalized patients are so harried that they give the impression of being disinterested in their clients. Patients feel that when a physician relates to them through a videotelephone, his emotional energies are not distracted by extraneous considerations and that he is totally devoted to them. During routine medical rounds, many physicians fail to look directly at their patients; they may focus on a leg, a student, or a wall. Because the picturephone forces the doctor to look at his patient, it enhances the physician-patient encounter (8).

Marshall McLuhan's contention that television represents "the most recent and spectacular electronic extension of the central nervous system" (9) has been given credence by Kenneth Bird's telemedicine project. In April of 1968 an interactive television (IATV) system was established that links the Massachusetts General Hospital to a health station in Boston's Logan Airport. (IATV differs from conventional television in that the sending and the receiving of audiovisual impulses are bidirectional rather than unidirectional.) Typically, a patient enters the Logan Airport health center and is greeted by a nurse-practitioner. By means of IATV, the patient engages in a dialogue with a physician located at the Massachusetts General Hospital. After acquiring a medical history, the doctor conducts a physical examination with the assistance of the nurse. For example, he has the nurse place a stethoscope over the patient's heart or chest, and the sounds are conveyed electronically from the patient to the physician. The health station has electrocardiogram and X-ray equipment; the resultant tracings and films can be transmitted to the doctor in a highly readable form. Blood smears can be magnified 1000 times, sent electronically, and visualized clearly by the physician. Even prescriptions can be conveyed from the hospital to the health station. Although the IATV uses black-and-white rather than color images, the high quality resolution of the picture allows the physician to make detailed observations of skin lesions and other aspects of surface anatomy (10–15).

With the exception of surgery, almost every medical specialty from dermatology to speech therapy to psychiatry has been practiced via IATV (15–16). Dr. Bird's telemedicine system can diagnose and treat 90 percent of the patients who present themselves to the Logan Airport health station. Furthermore, an independent assessment has shown that 85 percent of the patients were favorably disposed toward their telemedicine experiences (12). Not only were they receiving high quality medical care, they did not have to travel long distances and fight Boston traffic to obtain it. The system also has benefited doctors by providing educational programs and consultations. Ever since March 17, 1970, IATV has been used to provide "teleconsultations" from physicians at the Massachusetts General Hospital to their colleagues at the Bedford Veterans Administration Hospital. Bidirectional television can offer extensive diagnostic, therapeutic, and educational services at a reasonable expense; it costs only $75,000 to create two telemedicine centers located 20 to 40 miles apart (17).

IATV is being used throughout the nation. New York's Mount Sinai Hospital is providing pediatric care to East Harlem via bidirectional television (18). Since 1959 the University of Nebraska Medical Center has offered extensive neurological and psychological consultation, treatment, and education throughout the state. They even have been able to manage psychiatric units at the Norfolk State Mental Hospital, which is located 112 miles from the medical center. An entire statewide IATV medical network has been established to provide psychiatric and neurological services to three Veterans Administration hospitals (19).

A similar network has been created in Northern New England that links the medical centers of the University of Vermont and Dartmouth College with several community hospitals and a prison (20). Psychiatric consultations are provided routinely on a 24-hour-a-day basis from the Dartmouth-Hitchcock Mental Health Center to the Claremont General Hospital 26 miles away. Nonpsychiatric physicians in Claremont are able to observe these interviews and thereby enhance their psychiatric skills (21). Having conducted many of these consultations myself, I have been impressed that the television does not create an obstacle to the fulfillment of an intimate therapeutic encounter. For example, at the end of one session a patient totally forgot he was undergoing an electronic interview; he stood up and gratefully tried to shake the hand of the televised psychiatrist (20). Dr. Thomas Dwyer, a pioneer in the field, believes that telepsychiatry makes it easier for some patients to avail themselves of mental health services. He notes that while some clients avoid obtaining psychiatric help because they are frightened of hospital settings, others fear a direct meeting with a psychiatrist and prefer the less threatening accessibility afforded by televised therapy (22).

Telemedicine has also been provided in settings where health care services are often inferior. In July, 1973 telemedicine was introduced into several Miami jails by a team from the University of Miami School of Medicine, the Dade County Department of Hospitals, and Westinghouse Health Systems. Both black-and-white video and slow-scan color transmission have been utilized. (A slow-scan system can produce a still TV picture that can be conveyed electronically via regular telephone lines.) Although this project is only in its initial stages, it already appears to have raised the quality of medical services provided to the inmates (23).

The use of telephone lines to convey electrocardiograms, audio-response systems, phonovision, and interactive television are a few of the present-day medical applications of communication technology. Before projecting how these developments may be expanded upon in the future, a brief review of some of the advances in communications anticipated within the next 50 years may be useful.

COMMUNICATION TECHNOLOGY IN THE FUTURE. If the predictions of some communication experts materialize, in the future man's physical presence may give way to his electronic presence. This may occur through two predominant means. The first is through the extended use of the telephone, and the other is by the expanded use of television. Although a thorough discussion of these communication media is beyond the scope of this book, those aspects having particular relevance to the future of health care delivery are commented upon.

In 1945 there were fewer than 28 million telephones in the United States. By the end of 1973 this number had risen to more than 158 million. American Telephone and Telegraph estimates that by the outset of the 21st century this figure will climb to approximately 500 million. The use of the telephone will also expand qualitatively as well as quantitatively. International direct distance dialing will become available. The development of battery-operated lineless extension phones that will enable its users to place a call from wherever and whenever they choose are also anticipated. The recent invention of the wireless vest-pocket telephone represents a step in this direction (24).

Although the popularity of conventional telephones has

climbed dramatically, the public has been reluctant to embrace videotelephones. Originally introduced in 1964, a flurry of interest developed when they were demonstrated at the Union Carbide show the following year. In 1969 a dozen companies in Pittsburgh and later three others in Washington purchased the system. By 1974 all of these firms discontinued the service. In New York the Public Service Commission refused to approve the installation of videotelephones until conventional telephone service was improved. Nevertheless, A.T.&T. feels they are a marketable commodity and have accelerated their promotional efforts. In Chicago about 100 customers currently pay $87.50 a month plus installation and time charges for one set (25). In April of 1974 a visual conference phone system was established in two different cities that enabled six participants to conduct business as if they were sitting around the same meeting table. A spokesman for A.T.&T. told me that picturephones definitely will be available for hospital use by 1980. As videotelephones become more flexible, practical, and inexpensive, some authorities predict that by the year 2000 they will be as widely distributed as conventional telephones are today (26). It is anticipated that picturephones will be able to accommodate close-up and wide-angle views and thereby could visualize diagrams, patient charts, faculty meetings, and group therapy sessions (24).

Because the push button (Touch-Tone) telephone can function as a computer terminal, its increasing availability could bring a wide array of computerized services into the home. For example, if a woman wants to purchase a dress, she would not have to travel to a series of shops to find out what is available. Instead, she could dial her telephone and hear computerized inventories from a variety of stores. The possession of a personal computer terminal would also allow its owner to avail himself of a number of banking, educational, recreational, and business services. John Kemeny has predicted that by 1990 these automated services will be widely available in homes, schools, businesses, and hospitals (27). The telephone will function not only as a vehicle for conversation, but also as a medium for the exchange of computerized information.

The integration of computer and communication technology may be enhanced even further as progress is made in converting speech into a digital form. This development will allow the machine to "recognize" conversation. For example, if one wishes to find out how much is in his automated bank account, instead of having to press a number of telephone push buttons, he could inquire verbally (24). As computers are able to translate foreign languages, international communication may also be facilitated. Automated programs that translate Russian and Chinese into English have already been devised (28). If this ability is combined with the anticipated capacity of the computer to convert speech into digital form (29), language differences would no longer present a major obstacle to the worldwide exchange of information. These developments would move us one step closer to the implementation of the "global village" concept.

Future innovations in television technology may even exceed the intriguing possibilities envisioned by telephone and computer industries. Television's impact upon American society has been enormous. In 1973 there were more than 900 television stations in the United States. Ninety-six percent of American homes have at least one set, which operates on the average of six hours per day (30). As of March 1974, there were about 3070 cable television (CATV) systems offering programs to approximately 6150 communities and 8 million households in this country (31). Many believe that by 1980 a conventional television set will have between 20 and 40 channels (32). At least theoretically, this number could be increased to as many as 80 to 200 (33). We presently are unable to capitalize upon this potential because we lack the facilities for adequate broadband communication. Nevertheless, in the future co-axial cables, lasers, and communications satellites may be the major transmission vehicles for an expanded broadcasting capacity (27, 34-35). Conventional telephone wires could also be used to handle this increased load (36).

Interactive television will play an expanded role in the future. It has been estimated that by 1990 ninety percent of American homes will have IATV (37). Bidirectional television could provide the consumer with a wide range of services. Computer-assisted instruction, tutorial programs, and adult education courses could be offered via IATV. Business activities, such as secretarial aid, access to company files, computer-assisted meetings, and banking services could be made available. Information about medical and legal problems, current events (i.e., the electronic newspaper), transportation, ticket reservations, weather, and consumer goods also could be conveyed by IATV. Two-way television would allow people a greater selection of movies and theatrical productions and offer them up-to-date listings of local sporting and entertainment events. Many forms of interpersonal communication, such as message recordings and mail could be transmitted via IATV. If someone wants to examine the menues of several restaurants or to acquire access to library resources, they could simply turn on their television and receive this information. Experts claim that many of these services could be available on a limited basis by 1980 (38).

These services are considered to be performed by IATV because the viewer is able to select and interact with the program he receives. It is different from the IATV used in Bird's telemedicine project in that live moving images are not conveyed in both directions. Nevertheless, as the costs of television cameras decline, it is probable that lifelike pictures also could be transmitted from the home. In addition, the existence of communications satellites may allow for the global use of interactive television (17). IATV may alter the American way of life, just as unidirectional television has done so during the past two decades.

The capacity of television to present a three-dimensional image has been made possible by the use of holography. A holograph is a photographic record of an interface pattern between a reflected light wave from an object and a second wave of interfering light (35). The resultant effect is quite dramatic. Not only does the viewer observe the roundness of objects, but by moving his head from side to side he also can see around the object (24). It is anticipated that by 1983 three-dimensional unidirectional television will be commercially available (39). The realism afforded by holographic techniques will be enhanced even further as the size of the television image increases. Enlarging upon the picture tube to create full wall-sized TV would be impractical because the electronic equipment necessary to do so would occupy an inordinate amount of space. An alternative approach would be to use a projected image or to curve the wall as is done with Cinerama (24). By the year 2000 the typical American home could conceivably have a 3-D, full-wall sized interactive color television with stereophonic sound. A copying device could be attached to this complex audiovisual system to make permanent records of whatever comes over the screen (26).

ALTERNATIVE FUTURES IN MEDICAL COMMUNICATIONS. The anticipated developments in communication technology may have numerous implications for the future of health care delivery and of medical education. The effect that advanced communications will have upon the training and selection of medics is discussed in Chapter 7. For now, however, an overview of the modifications that the communications revolution may bring to the provision of medical services is examined. Not all of the possibilities will necessarily materialize within the next 50 years, but the potential for many of these developments to occur is highly plausible, and therefore, they are worth considering.

The widespread availability of videotelephones, IATV, and computer terminals within the home may allow patients to receive a large proportion of their medical care without having to travel to a hospital, clinic, or office. A patient may give his medical history to a clinician over a videophone or an interactive television. Because the practitioner is able to see as well as to hear the patient, many aspects of the physical examination could be performed by remote control. While the patient remains at home, his physiological parameters could be measured by wireless sensing devices. Already the Boeing Company has created a small battery-powered unit to monitor a patient's temperature, blood pressure, pulse, and electrocardiogram. Upon a radio command from a central station, physiologic data on the patient are sent by the transmitter and printed out for the clinician (24). As the cost of this unit or one like it declines, people who would benefit from owning such a device could purchase them for home use. Cardiac patients will be able to obtain inexpensive EKG leads which could be inserted into a conventional telephone outlet. After the patient is taught how to attach the electrodes to his body, the electrical impulses from his heart could be sent via telephone wires to a central computer for analysis. In the near future fashion-conscious patients will be able to purchase filigree bracelets and necklaces that contain minute monitoring devices and compartments for holding medications. If the wearer's cardiac rate becomes abnormally accelerated or irregular, a buzzer is sounded. The jewelry has small compartments that hold corrective medications which could be used by the patient when the alarm beeps. A pendant that monitors air pollution and holds a 10-minute emergency oxygen supply has been designed for asthma, hay-fever, and other respiratory disease sufferers. It also has a protective face mask for use when the buzzer signals (40).

Under a medic-computer model, the patient may respond to medical history questions flashed on a videophone or an IATV by pushing the appropriate buttons on his Touch-Tone telephone. In many circumstances the patient's medical requirements could be met without him ever having to leave his home. Medical information derived from the patient could be analyzed by a central computer, and the medic could discuss the results with the patient and suggest treatment via a telecommunications linkup. Only if certain aspects of the physical examination cannot be performed by remote control or if selected ancillary tests are needed, would the patient have to go to a regional health center.

Many patients miss the vanishing tradition of the doctor's house call. As the practice of medicine became more sophisticated, the physician required the use of complex equipment that was either too bulky or too expensive to carry around with him. These *apparati medica* could be situated only in the physician's office or in a hospital. Patients had to leave their homes to acquire the benefits of these sophisticated devices. For the doctor to spend hours fighting traffic to visit a patient's home became a highly uneconomical practice. Thus, the house call has all but disappeared. In the future, however, the expanded use of communication technology may resurrect the institution of the home visit, albeit in an unique historical form. The electronic house call may be a common occurrence in an era where videotelephones, IATV, sensing devices, and computer terminals are found in the typical American dwelling (41).

Because geographic proximity could be replaced by electronic proximity, future psychotherapists and their patients could sit in their respective homes and participate in a therapeutic dialog. Group therapy could be performed by using a conference videophone, just as corporation executives presently use the conference telephone to discuss business. "Teleprescriptions" could be conveyed via interactive television and copied by the patient in his home (12). Because ambulatory psychiatric treatment requires a minimal amount of sophisticated instrumentation, the use of communication technology may all but replace outpatient psychiatric clinics. Similarly, the use of IATV and videophones may decrease the need for psychiatric hospitals. Currently, many patients are admitted because their families or friends are unable to provide them with adequate supervision (42). In the future, however, the monitoring of patient behavior at home could occur with the aid of advanced telecommunications. Although this increased capacity to supervise patients within their home environment will not eliminate the need for psychiatric hospitals, it could go a long way in this direction. *

Many experts have suggested that if the life span of the populace increases without a concomitant reduction in the deleterious effects of aging, the need for nursing homes will escalate dramatically. Many of these repositories of the aged are excessively populated and inadequately staffed (43). Both of these problems may be partially overcome with the assistance of advanced telecommunications. Many patients who today require the supervision of a nursing home may in the future obtain these services in their homes by the electronic observation of their behavior.

* The decreasing utilization of inpatient facilities began in the mid 1950s with the introduction of effective psychoactive drugs and a greater focus upon community approaches to the treatment of mental disease (42). In the future new discoveries in psychotherapeutics will dovetail with developments in telecommunications to diminish even further the use of psychiatric hospitals.

These projections should not be equated with Kafkaesque images of an omnipresent Big Brother, nor should they imply the advancing specter of dehumanized medical care. The use of electronic monitoring would be voluntary and would be done with the full acknowledgement of those being observed. The patient could obtain privacy simply by turning off his television or videophone. Many patients could remain in their dwellings instead of being sequestered in the unfamiliar and often frightening environment of the old-age home. Furthermore, money presently spent for institutional care could be used by the elderly in more fulfilling ways.

Undoubtedly, some of the aged will still need to live in nursing homes. The problem of overburdened or undertrained staffs may be minimized by electronically introducing additional staff and medical expertise via a telecommunication system. For example, if a patient has a sudden heart attack, instead of having to wait for an ambulance to come and bring the patient to the hospital to see a physician, a telemedicine system could provide immediate consultation.

The expanded use of wireless sensing devices for high-risk cardiac patients may help reduce even further the critical time between the onset of a heart attack and its subsequent treatment. One of the major difficulties with many present day chronic care institutions is that, although they generally need a lower staff-to-patient ratio than do acute general hospitals, they require the continuous and immediate availability of the sophisticated staff and equipment of the acute general hospital. Some authorities have suggested that chronic care facilities be situated adjacent to acute general hospitals (43). Unfortunately, often this property is expensive and unavailable. Therefore, chronic care institutions are usually located far away from the sources of acute medical care. In the future, however, telecommunications could replace the need for geographic proximity with electronic proximity, and full-time emergency treatment could be available to chronic care facilities without the necessity of being situated near an acute general hospital (41).

The establishment of a complex telecommunication and computer network may also facilitate the provision of medical care to communities that presently receive inadequate services. The problems of recruiting practitioners to certain urban and rural areas has been well documented (44). The lack of medical services in some locales is one of the major deficiencies in our contemporary health care system. The greater use of economic incentives, the establishment of a national medical service corps, and the development of health maintenance organizations are a few of the proposals that have been advanced to alleviate this problem (43, 45). The greater use of communication technology in the future may partially solve the dilemmas that arise from the maldistribution of health care personnel. Because electronic presence could substitute for physical presence, telecommunications systems could deliver medical services to understaffed rural communities and urban ghettos. Tentative progress in this area already has been made. The further development of these telecommunication programs would enable every citizen to obtain health care, regardless of geographical considerations. The decreasing costs of equipment and the increasing use of co-axial cables, lasers, and telephone wires for bidirectional audiovisual transmission may allow for the widespread use of telecommunications for health care delivery within the next 25 to 50 years. If so, a practitioner may no longer be necessary in every area or in every community for comprehensive medical services to exist.

The growing use of communication satellites (COMSAT) may one day result in the internationalization of health care delivery. Whether for an earache in Africa or a malignancy in Asia, practitioners on the opposite side of the world could diagnose and treat the disorder with the assistance of communication and computer technology. Although IATV can already be transmitted via COMSAT (17), the capacity to offer global medical care could take at least another four to five decades before it is developed. Other difficulties would have to be resolved to maximize the internationalization of medical care services. Computers would have to be programmed specially in consideration of the differing prevalences of diseases in varying parts of the world. Language problems would have to be overcome. The use of automated

language translaters (28–29) or of an international language, such
as Esperanto, may alleviate this obstacle. Possibly the greatest
barriers to the implementation of internationalized medical care
delivery would be financial, cultural, and technical. Nevertheless,
the emergence of a world wide IATV or videophone network will
eventually materialize, and when it does it could dramatically
alter global health care activities.

Underlying this brief survey of the alternative ways by which
communication technology may affect medicine's future is a
fundamental but infrequently recognized consideration. We often
confuse the *meaning* of mobility with the *means* of mobility. We
forget that an essential purpose of human movement is to avail
ourselves of a new or at least a different array of sensory stimuli
(46). We no longer have to go to a stadium to see a football game;
a television can bring the stadium to us. More than ever before
communication technology is able to transport us from experience
to experience, and as it does so, some of us find ourselves prefer-
ring the electronic experience over the real one (47). Television
has replaced legitimate theatre and films as a major source of
entertainment. Many sports fans prefer watching a game on
television to attending one in person. These trends suggest that
physical mobility may be giving way to electronic mobility.
According to the Stanford Research Institute, in terms of dollar
volume in the United States, the communication industry will
overtake the transportation industry by the end of this decade
(46). Thus, when considering and planning for medicine's long-
range future, we will need to take into account that telemobility
may increasingly replace physical movement. The communications revolution may permeate all aspects of human experience.
Undoubtedly, it will alter where we live, how we live, and possibly
—just possibly—why we live.

These issues are not raised for the sake of mere philosophical
speculation. When designing the future, health care planners
must consider the psychological implications of man's preference
for electronic experiences. If taken to its logical extreme, the

unrestrained use of computer and communication technology would so radically transform civilization that inevitably society would consist of people living in isolated cubicles who would never directly encounter nature or one another. Although I assume that this frightening prospect will never materialize, it underscores a basic problem that may inhibit the extensive deployment of advanced telecommunications. People will not choose to live in a technological fortress; they still will attend the theatre, stroll in the country, dance at a party, and play cards with the neighbors. Although IATV could save women an inordinate amount of time shopping, they may prefer to spend these "wasted" hours going from store to store just for the sake of getting out of their homes and meeting other people. Similarly, despite the numerous conveniences telecommunications could offer patients, many individuals will still want to see their clinicians in person. Although telecommunications will significantly alter the future delivery of medical services, it will never completely replace face-to-face encounters between patients and practitioners.

NOTES

1. Freed, R. N. (1967). "Legal Aspects of Computer Use in Medicine." *Law and Contemporary Problems*, 32:674–706.

2. Stehling, K. R. (1972). *Computers and You*. New York: New American Library.

3. Allen, S. I., and M. Otten (1969). "The Telephone As A Computer Input-Output Terminal for Medical Information." *Journal of the American Medical Association*, 208:673–679.

4. DeLeo, J. M., W. C. White, and D. Songco (1972). "Medical Audio Response Telecommunication Information Network." *Bio-Medical Computing*, 3:293–305.

5. Plexico, P. S. (1972). "Computer Driven Voice Response in Medical Applications." Mimeo.

6. Stockbridge, C. D. (1972). "The Performance of Picturephone Systems in Transmitting Medical Data." In W. C. Zarnstorff, W. R. Hendee, and P. L. Carson (eds.), *Application of Optical Instrumentation in Medicine*. Chicago: Society of Photo-Optical Instrumentation Engineers. Pp. 9–16.

7. *American Medical News* (1973). "Picturephone Saving Steps in Hospital," 16(35):19.

8. Bush, I. M. "A Ten Station Picturephone System in the Modern Delivery of Urologic Care." Mimeo.

9. McLuhan, M., and Q. Fiore (1967). *The Medium Is the Message.* New York: Bantam.

10. Bird, K. T. (1973). "Conclusions from Experiences with Telemedicine." Paper read at the Second Arizona Conference on Rural Health, Tucson, Arizona. April 30.

11. Murphy, R. L. H., P. Block, K. T. Bird, and P. Yurchak (1973). "Accuracy by Cardiac Auscultation by Microwave." *Chest,* 63:578–581.

12. Murphy, R. L. H., Jr., G. L. Cohen, J. Herskovits, and K. T. Bird. "Tele-Diagnosis: A New Community Health Resource. I. Observations on the Feasibility of Tele-Diagnosis Based on 1000 Patient Transactions." Mimeo.

13. Bird, K. T. (1972). "Cardiopulmonary Frontiers: Quality Health Care Via Interactive Television." *Chest,* 61:204–205.

14. Andrus, W. S., and K. T. Bird (1972). "Teleradiology: Evolution Through Bias to Reality." *Chest,* 62:655–657.

15. Bird, K. T., M. H. Clifford, and T. F. Dwyer (1971). *Teleconsultation: A New Health Information Exchange System.* Unpublished report.

16. Dwyer, T. F. (1973). "Telepsychiatry: Psychiatric Consultation by Interactive Television." *American Journal of Psychiatry,* 130:865–869.

17. Bird, K. T. (1973). "Telemedicine: Medicine of the Future Today." Lowell Lecture delivered at the Massachusetts Eye and Ear Infirmary, Boston. March 27.

18. *New York Times* (1973). "Child Clinic Gets Physicians Via TV." June 7. Section C, p. 34.

19. Wittson, C. L., and R. Benschoter (1972). "Two-Way Television: Helping the Medical Center Reach Out." *American Journal of Psychiatry,* 129:624–627.

20. Thorne, B. K. (1973). "Medical Care Via Television." *Dartmouth Alumni Magazine,* 65(April):18–21.

21. Solow, C., R. J. Weiss, B. J. Bergen, and C. J. Sanborn (1971). "24-Hour Psychiatric Consultation Via TV." *American Journal of Psychiatry,* 127:1684–1687.

22. *Footnotes to the Future* (1974). "Medical Notes," 4(5):2–3.

23. Hartley, E. (1975). "Quality Care for Prison Patients." *Prism,* 3(4):34–41.

24. Hellman, H. (1969). *Communications In the World of the Future.* New York: Evans.

25. *New York Times* (1974). "Picturephones," March 31. P. 33.

26. *Wall Street Journal* (1967). *Here Comes Tomorrow!: Living and Working in the Year 2000.* Princeton, N. J.: Dow Jones Books.

27. Kemeny, J. G. (1972). *Man and the Computer.* New York: Scribner's.

28. Fink, D. G. (1966). *Computers and the Human Mind.* Garden City, N. J.: Doubleday.

29. Winograd, T. (1974). "When Will Computers Understand People?" *Psychology Today*, 7(12):73–79.

30. Thompson, T. (1973). "Telecommunications As A Potential Health Education Tool." *Journal of Medical Education*, 48:1155–1156.

31. *Footnotes to the Future* (1974). "Media Notes: Cable TV Facts," 4(7)3.

32. Flagler, J. M. (1972). "The Flight from the Shlockhouse." *Intellectual Digest*, 3(3):24–26.

33. Bagdikian, B. H. (1971). "How Much More Communication Can We Stand?" *The Futurist*, 5:180–183.

34. Miller, A. R. (1971). *The Assault on Privacy: Computers, Data Banks, and Dossiers.* New York: New American Library.

35. Kahn, H., and A. J. Wiener (1967). *Toward the Year 2000: A Framework for Speculation.* New York: Macmillan.

36. Wedemeyer, C. A. (1967). "The Future of Educational Technology in the U.S.A." In G. Moir (ed.), *Teaching and Television: ETV Explained.* Oxford: Pergamon. Pp. 132–157.

37. Jones, M. V. (1973). "How Cable Television May Change Our Lives." *The Futurist*, 7:196–199.

38. Baran, P. (1973). "30 Services That Two-Way Television Can Provide." *The Futurist*, 7:202–210.

39. Edelhart, M. (1973). "3D TV Is Coming." *TV Guide*, 21(50):13–15.

40. *Footnotes to the Future* (1974). "Technology Notes: Medical Jewelry," 4(8):4.

41. Maxmen, J. S. (1974). "Communications, Medicine and the Future." Paper delivered at the Western Psychiatric Institute and Clinic, Pittsburgh. January 7.

42. Maxmen, J. S., G. J. Tucker, and M. D. LeBow (1974). *Rational Hospital Psychiatry: The Reactive Environment.* New York: Brunner/Mazel.

43. Chase, A. (1971). *The Biological Imperatives: Health, Politics, and Human Survival.* Baltimore: Penguin.

44. Mason, H. R. (1972). "Manpower Needs by Specialty." *Journal of the American Medical Association*, 219:1621–1626.

45. Mechanic, D. (1972). *Public Expectations and Health Care: Essays on the Changing Organization of Health Services.* New York: Wiley-Interscience.

46. *Kaiser Aluminum News* (1966). "Ballet of the Clockwork Dinosaurs," 24(3):6–17.

47. *Kaiser Aluminum News* (1966). "Riders of the Electronic Surf," 24(3): 18–30.

5

THE HEALTH PROFESSIONS_____

By illustrating the potential effect that technological, social, and psychological factors will exert on the future delivery of health care services, I have suggested that these forces inevitably will lead to the gradual obsolescence of the physician. The impact of historical change, however, will not be limited to a single profession; everyone of the health care occupations will be affected. These transformations will significantly shape medicine's future, and they will alter the career lives of about one out of every 25 Americans between the ages of 18 and 65. As Table 2 documents, about 4.3 million people currently are employed in a wide diversity of health-related fields (1). Rather than examine all of these professions (an exhaustive undertaking), I concentrate on those occupations I believe will either play a major role in the medicine of tomorrow or will be greatly influenced by anticipated historical developments. I do not discuss the future activities of doctors in this chapter because this topic has already been explored.

TABLE II.   ESTIMATED NUMBER OF HEALTH CARE
PROFESSIONALS IN 1971 (1)

Health Field	Number
1. Nursing and Related Services	2,072,500
2. Medicine and Osteopathy	334,000
3. Secretarial and Office Services	287,500
4. Dentistry and Allied Services	265,700
5. Environmental Health	243,500
6. Clinical Laboratory Services	150,500
7. Pharmacy	140,750
8. Radiologic Technology	87,500
9. Medical Records	54,500
10. Basic Health Sciences	51,200
11. Administration	48,400
12. Dietetic and Nutritional Services	37,000
13. Optometry and Opticianry	35,200
14. Social Work	29,800
15. Psychology	27,000
16. Food and Drug Protective Services	24,100
17. Physical Therapy	24,000
18. Health Education	22,500
19. Speech Pathology and Audiology	22,000
20. Chiropractic and Naturopathy	16,500
21. Vocational Rehabilitation Counselling	14,800
22. Occupational Therapy	13,500
23. Health Information and Communication	11,550
24. Specialized Rehabilitation Services	11,300
25. Biomedical Engineering	10,800
26. Medical Library Services	7,900
27. Podiatry	7,100
28. Midwifery	4,950
29. Orthotic and Prosthetic Technology	3,600
30. Automatic Data Processing	2,500
31. Anthropology and Sociology	1,600
32. Health and Vital Statistics	1,350
33. Economic Health Research	400
34. Miscellaneous Health Services	321,800
Totals	4,387,300

NURSING. The nursing profession is in the midst of an identity crisis. Although the phrase *identity crisis* has become so overused that its potency has been weakened and its definition blurred (2), I have chosen to apply this description with a specific meaning in mind. The dilemmas of the profession are serious, but more importantly I want to convey the Eriksonian notion of an identity crisis: ". . . a necessary turning point, a crucial moment, when development must move one way or another, marshaling resources of growth, recovery, and further differentiation. . . . (which can result from) the tensions of rapid historical change" (2, p. 16). Because I believe that nursing is experiencing this kind of an identity crisis, I suspect that they, among all of the occupations discussed in this chapter, will undergo the most dramatic changes in the future. To understand these changes, we must examine the current problems of the nursing profession.

Present Dilemmas. Nursing is a diverse collection of professionals, rather than a single occupational group. This amalgam of professionals receives highly varied training and conducts widely dissimilar functions. Basically, they can be divided into two groups: technical nurses who perform routine clinical activities and professional nurses who assume educational, administrative, and more complex clinical responsibilities.

Three-year diploma nurses were the first to emerge in the United States. Originally, most of their education was practical, rather than academic, with approximately 97 per cent of their time devoted to bedside nursing. In exchange for food, lodging, and minimal training, these students provided a cheap source of labor for American hospitals. In the late-1920s, seventy-three percent of hospitals with nursing schools employed no graduate nurses; they relied completely upon students, who received approximately 10 percent of the salary of graduate nurses. This apprenticeship system failed to provide nurses with adequate scientific backgrounds. Thus, over the objections of fiscal-conscious hospital administrators, four-year university-trained baccalaureate-degree nursing programs were established.

Unlike the diploma courses, the four-year programs stressed general education and the study of science and minimized on-the-job training. Today the first two years of these programs generally consist of a liberal arts education, and the last two years are devoted primarily to nursing theory, with only brief interludes of clinical experience. In 1952 two-year associate-degree programs were created; they also emphasize classroom teaching rather than bedside nursing. Since then Masters and Ph.D. degrees have been granted to nurses who wish either to pursue an academic or an administrative career or to assume highly sophisticated clinical duties. Over the years an academic focus in which theoretical knowledge is stressed has replaced the apprenticeship system, with its emphasis on practical skills (3–4).

Licensed Practical Nurses (LPNs) and attendants have assumed the vast majority of mundane nursing chores such as changing bed pans and washing patients. Recently, as registered nurses (RNs) have been performing more sophisticated administrative, educational, and clinical tasks, many LPNs have been executing the former duties of RNs, such as dispensing medications. As a result, LPNs have been conducting more significant clinical functions, while attendants, aides, and orderlies have been performing elementary nursing chores.

Registered nurses have become increasingly vocal in expressing their professional grievances. Low pay, erratic hours, limited career mobility, inferior status, minimal responsibility, and sexism have been some of their more frequently mentioned complaints (3, 5–6). This discontent has contributed to a serious attrition rate among nurses. One out of every four nurses is totally inactive; another 25 percent are active only to the extent of maintaining licensure. Of the remaining 50 percent almost one out of three works part time. Even among those who are full time, many perform nonpatient care activities, such as teaching and administrating. Furthermore, approximately one-third of all students who enter nursing schools drop out before graduation (3). As a result, in 1970 there was an estimated shortage of 150,000 nurses in the United States, and this figure had risen to about 200,000 by 1975* (4). This shortage is not due to a lack of educated nurses, but rather to a disparity between the optimistic expectations and the disheartening realities of a nursing career.

This disillusionment, and the nursing shortages that emerge from it, will lead to four major trends: (a) LPNs will increasingly assume tasks formerly performed by RNs (8). (b) Three-year diploma programs will be phased out. According to one estimate, in 1956 there were 26,828 graduates of three-year programs; by 1980 there will be only 5,118 graduates. Another projection suggests that diploma programs will disappear altogether by as early as 1978 (4). (c) As the number of hospital-based diploma programs decline, university-based baccalaureate- and associate-degree programs will increase. Conservative estimates predict that by 1980 there will be 15,932 baccalaureate- and 27,911 associate-degree graduates. This would constitute, since 1969, a 90 percent increase of baccalaureate-degree graduates and a 221 percent increase of associate-degree graduates (4). (d) Whereas the training of clinical nurses was once the responsibility of technically oriented diploma nurses, recently this function has been taken over by those who have master's degrees or higher (5). Collectively, these trends demonstrate a gradual change of emphasis from clinical to academic nursing. This development partially reflects the decade in which it gained momentum. For the 1960s was a period in which education was viewed as a remedy to whatever problems ailed a particular individual, profession, or society. Upon more sober reflection, however, this naive faith in the academe has not been fulfilled.

The shift from hospital- to university-based programs has resulted in serious problems and unfortunate realignments emerging within the nursing profession. Of the 700,000 practicing nurses fewer than 3 percent have a master's or higher degree. Nevertheless, this educational elite is the official spokesman for the

---

* Although one hears a great deal about a severe doctor shortage, the present nursing shortage is more than three times that of physicians (7).

entire profession. Sequestered in academia they often are unfamiliar with the daily problems of the 579,000 clinically oriented diploma graduates who constitute the bulk of nursing personnel. As a result, there is a serious schism between nursing education and nursing service (5). This problem not only exists over matters of official policy, but also in the area of training. Because higher-degree programs involve only a minimal amount of direct patient contact, their graduates are ill-equipped to provide clinical training. It is difficult to supervise and teach clinical skills without adequate practical experience. Nurses themselves are acutely aware of this deficiency. A study of why 66 baccalaureate nursing students sought paid part-time and summer jobs revealed that they *all* did so primarily to acquire clinical experience and professional self-confidence (9). Without this exposure, many university-trained nurses are thrust into positions of responsibility for which they have been inadequately prepared (5). Graduates who enter hospital nursing discover quickly that their academic training, at best, has poorly equipped them to perform clinical activities, and at worst, has been a total waste of time. As Sadler, Sadler, and Bliss have observed:

> Why teach the nurse anatomy, physiology, chemistry, anthropology, microbiology, the signs and symptoms of disease, the course of and response to medications, and other therapeutic procedures, as well as the possible outcome and complications, if she is unable to utilize this information in ways which directly improve the patient's health? If the nurse, as suggested by some, should only collect data and make observations, then a brief course in interviewing is all that is needed. Why teach pharmacology now that the pharmacy in many hospitals prepares the proper dosages in separate packages and the nurse may only deliver them to the patient? Why take the long time to fill the nurse's head with signs and symptoms of disease if diagnosis is not to be her function? To what avail is physiology and anatomy if the nurse may only sponge it, roll it over, or assist it out of bed (5, pp. 58–59)?

As the authors imply, a scholarly education is unnecessary to perform traditional nursing chores; these tasks can and are increasingly being conducted by LPNs. Furthermore, as Sadler *et al.* suggest, baccalaureate nurses who work in hospitals are confronted immediately with the disparity between the expectations and the realities of a nursing career. No wonder the turnover rate among staff nurses in American hospitals is over 70 percent, while among elementary and secondary school teachers—also predominately female and from the same socioeconomic background—the turnover rate is approximately 20 percent (10).

If clinically oriented baccalaureate nurses are to capitalize upon their academic experiences, they must acquire further training to become nurse-practitioners or nurse-clinicians. Usually, a nurse-practitioner is an RN who receives an additional six months of didactic training to enable her to provide general medical care in an ambulatory setting. A nurse-clinician has at least a master's degree and, under the supervision of a physician, performs complex medical tasks in cardiac and intensive care units or provides diagnostic and treatment services in specialty areas, such as pediatrics, obstetrics, gynecology, and psychiatry. By assuming these responsibilities, both groups hope to obtain from their work a new sense of professionalism, independence, and dignity. However, they may become disillusioned.

Freidson has observed that professions differ from occupations in that the former has ultimate control in determining and applying the skills of the trade (11). Regardless of the sophistication of their training or the initials following their names, most clinically oriented nurses practice under the auspices of physicians. If we accept Freidson's distinction between professions and occupations, doctors belong to the former, while nurses belong to the latter. *

Many nurses who would aspire to be independent practitioners object to being controlled by doctors (6, 12–13). They argue that because of their training and "professionalism" they ought to be free of physician domination and be allowed to render clinical decisions independent of the doctor. Nevertheless, the fact is that some individual ultimately must be in charge of a patient's care. Although admittedly some nurses are more knowledgeable and

---

* For literary convenience I have not made this distinction in the text and, therefore, have used the terms *profession* and *occupation* interchangeably.

resourceful than some physicians, for the most part the latter are better equipped to coordinate and to make critical decisions affecting a patient's treatment. Thus, for the nurse to practice independently of the physician is usually neither possible nor desirable. This conviction is not stated with the intent of denigrating the utility of highly trained nurses; it is an attempt to underscore the futility of their striving to practice autonomously.

If a totally independent relationship between nurses and doctors is untenable, a totally dependent relationship is equally undesirable. The latter fails to capitalize upon the training and skills of baccalaureate nurses and tends to relegate them to the role of glorified servants. The ongoing debate over the relationship of nurses to physicians has tended to polarize those who advocate total independence and those who favor total dependence. However, there is a realistic and constructive middle ground: Nurses and doctors are dependent upon one another. Because physicians cannot practice without nurses and vice versa, nurses should play an *interdependent* role as a member of the health care team (5). This interdependent role can be maximized, if they function as nurse-practitioners or nurse-clinicians. In these capacities they will be able to take advantage of the highly specialized education they have received.

Like physician's assistants, nurse-practitioners and nurse-clinicians assume major clinical duties under the supervision of a doctor. One might ask why baccalaureate nurses do not become trained as physician's assistants. In 1970 the executive director of the AMA unilaterally announced a plan whereby 100,000 nurses would become physician's assistants. The president of the American Nurses' Association (ANA) quickly condemned the proposal, stating that it would further deplete the supply of nurses. She also seemed to resent any unilateral action of the AMA that affected the nursing profession. When nurses were striving to enhance their independence from doctors, the suggestion that they should become physician's assistants served only to raise the specter of further medical domination (5). Failing to recognize the interdependent relationship between nurses and doctors, the notion that the former should become assistants to the latter was distasteful to the ANA. As a result of the AMA's tactless diplomacy and the ANA's obsession with occupational boundaries, we have inherited a bizarre situation wherein nurse-practitioners, nurse-clinicians, and physician's assistants perform similar functions, but receive varied educational experiences and maintain different professional identities, organizations, and titles. This meaningless pluralism will have to be overcome, if rationality, cohesiveness, and coherence are to be brought to bear upon future health care delivery systems.

Future Directions. To speak of the future of the nursing pro-fession*s*, rather than of the nursing profession, would be more accurate. Contemporary nursing consists of a conglomerate of occupations, with each constituent group having its own clinical responsibilities and training experiences (14). Rather than discuss every nursing category, I will simplify matters by projecting the futures of technical and professional nurses.

Technical nurses (associate, diploma, LPNs, attendants, order-lies, and aides) may continue to assume a greater proportion of routine bedside nursing and ward administration tasks. Computers probably will assist them in the performance of these duties by automatically assigning rooms, obtaining medical records, keeping track of medications, and so on (15). Despite the radical changes expected to occur in medicine's future, routine bedside nursing may undergo the *least* modification. Regardless of the model of health care delivery, there always will be a need for technical nursing. As professional nurses assume more complicated duties, recruiting and, more importantly, retaining technical nurses will be necessary. If the appalling turnover rate among technical nurses is to be reduced, they will, at a minimum, need to be offered greater financial inducements and more reasonable work-ing hours. Moreover, a fundamental realignment in the political structure of the nursing profession may be useful. Instead of the present system, whereby upper-echelon professional nurses issue mandates affecting technical nurses, for technical nurses to have leaders and teachers who come from their own ranks may be preferable. If this would occur, it would put an end to the mythology that there is a single nursing profession. If the spokesmen, supervisors, and educators of technical nurses were to be drawn from the ranks of technical, rather than from professional nursing, the former would probably have a more responsive leadership. Although this alternative future may be desirable, it hardly is inevitable. The professional nursing elite may jealously guard its authority and would be unlikely to abdicate this power. Similarly, lower-echelon technical nurses, with their characteristic passivity, generally have been unwilling to demand a larger voice in the conduct of their own affairs. Nevertheless, with concerted efforts on the part of technical nurses, they could exercise greater control over their own professional destinies.

Professional nurses (Ph.D., masters, and baccalaureate) can be expected to undergo significant structural and functional modifications over the next 50 years. Although the exact nature of these changes is difficult to predict, several viable alternate futures exist. Under a health-team model, clinically oriented professional nurses could function as physician's assistants, but retain their identities as nurse-practitioners or as nurse-clinicians. This would represent a continuation of the status quo. Although clinically oriented nurses could maintain their professional identities, another alternative would be that they abandon their nursing affiliation and become physician's assistants. If they are to function as physician's assistants, why not *be* physician's assistants? Why take from four to eight years of education to become nurse-practitioners or nurse-clinicians, when training to do identical tasks as physician's assistants can be accomplished within one to three years? They still could retain their interdependent relationship to other members of the medical team. Furthermore, why have a series of health care personnel who perform similar functions? Admittedly, given the tendency of professions to perpetuate themselves, clinically oriented professional nurses probably will not render themselves obsolete by joining the ranks of physician's assistants. Nevertheless, common sense and idealism, reinforced by intelligent private and government funding, could bring an end to this antiquated pluralism.

Under a medic-computer model, nurse-practitioners, nurse-clinicians, or physician's assistants would no longer be needed to perform patient care activities. During the transition from a health-team to a medic-computer model, professional or technical nurses who wish to provide clinical services could become medics. In a Post-Physician Era the need to train and retain clinically oriented professional nurses would become unnecessary. A more logical career path would be to be trained directly as a medic, rather than detour via the route of nursing

The future of educationally oriented professional nurses may take a different course from their clinical counterparts. Although I believe it would be less than desirable, professional nurses will probably continue to train technical nurses. Because technical nurses will be needed under both a health-team and a medic-computer model, professional nursing educators probably will have an important role to play for many years to come. During the transition from a health-team to a medic-computer model, nursing educators could use their academic experiences to train medics. Once a medic-computer model is fully actualized, professional nursing educators will no longer need to train nurse-practitioners and nurse-clinicians, because these personnel would be unnecessary in a Post-Physician Era. In the 21st century nursing educators will continue to perform significant duties, albeit on a more limited basis. Of course, on the unlikely possibility that technical nurses choose their leaders and teachers from their own ranks, professional nurses who specialize in education would be without any meaningful activities to perform. If so, like the physician, higher-echelon nurses would be rendered obsolete. Although this possibility is unlikely, we must remember that ever since the days of Florence Nightingale the nursing profession has undergone dramatic changes. And if there is one thing we know about the future, it is that change is inevitable.

THE PHYSICIAN'S ASSISTANT. Although doctors have been conspicuously disinterested in the internal machinations of the nursing profession, they have been passionately vocal about the physician's assistant (PA). To some he represents the worst of the past, while to others he constitutes the wave of the future. The extent to which either view prevails will partially influence future systems of health care delivery. Therefore, in projecting anticipated developments within medicine, we must examine the present condition and future potential of the physician's assistant.

The concept of the physician's assistant originated in 18th-century Russia where feldshers have become a cadre of "medical workers" who assist urban physicians in the performance of technical duties and assume preventive medicine and environmental control responsibilities in rural settings (16).

The idea of using physician's assistants did not receive serious consideration in the United States until 1961. Recognizing the nation's doctor shortage, Charles Hudson suggested the creation of a new class of health care professional "who could not only handle many technical procedures but could also take some degree of medical responsibility" (17). Since then Dr. Hudson's proposal has generated a flurry of professional and public interest. Many hoped that physician's assistants would alleviate the alleged doctor shortage; be fiscally sound, because PAs would require a shorter period of training than doctors; capitalize upon the skills of discharged military corpsmen; save consumers money because they could receive medical services from less expensive PAs;* provide increased primary, preventive, and emergency care; offer higher quality and more dignified medical services, because patients would not have to rely as much upon overburdened physicians; and permit doctors to concentrate on more specialized tasks (3).

With these expectations, Duke University launched the first American physician's assistant training program in 1965 (20). Although nine years later there were only 1800 graduates practicing in the United States, more than 70 training programs currently are producing about 1000 graduates annually (18, 21). These students are coming from a large pool of individuals, including 7000 fully qualified medical school applicants who each

---

* Whereas the average annual salary for a PA is between $10,000 to $15,000 (18), the typical doctor earns between $34,500 to $62,000 per year (19).

year fail to get accepted because of limited space, 700,000 active and 650,000 retired registered nurses, medical corpsmen who return to civilian life, college graduates who wish to be in the health field without undergoing the rigors of medical school, and other health care personnel (e.g., pharmacists, inhalation therapists, laboratory technologists, aides) (3, 22).

Both executive and congressional branches of government have supported the establishment of PA programs. Because of the doctor shortage, the public interest in the PA concept, the large pool of potential applicants, and the endorsement of most politicians, there would appear to be few obstacles to the widespread deployment of physician's assistants.

Nevertheless, several problems have emerged which may limit their utilization. These factors include conflicts over the extent of their medical abilities, their uncertain legal status, their relationship to nursing, and their acceptance by physicians and patients (3, 16, 21–25). Although originally PAs were expected to function primarily as general practitioners in locales that were deprived of medical services, this prospect has not been fully realized. Many PAs are locating in relatively prosperous areas because their pay demands are not being met by rural communities. Others are choosing to work with specialists rather than affiliate with primary care physicians (20). Because PAs are employed by doctors, they are establishing patterns of practice that resemble those of physicians. *

Like physicians, PAs are expected to meet with an individual

---

* Having recognized this development, the National Academy of Sciences has classified PAs into three categories. The Type A assistant ". . .is distinguished by his ability to integrate and interpret (clinical) findings on the basis of general medical knowledge and to exercise a degree of independent judgment. The Type B assistant, while not equipped with general knowledge and skills relative to the whole range of medical care, possesses exceptional skill in one clinical specialty. . . .The Type C assistant is capable of performing a variety of (general clinical) tasks. . .although he does not possess the level of medical knowledge necessary to integrate and interpret findings. He is similar to a Type A assistant in the number of areas in which he can perform, but he cannot exercise the degree of independent synthesis and judgment of which Type A is capable" (26, p. 3–4).

patient, acquire a history, conduct a physical examination, order ancillary tests, and so on. Functioning in this manner is necessary if PAs are to be hired by and form a compatible working relationship with their employing physicians. In the future, however, as computer technology exerts a greater influence upon the delivery of clinical services, the activities of physician's assistants may be altered. For example, they may perform like those allied health personnel who work at the Kaiser-Permanente multiphasic screening program. These allied health professionals guide and coordinate the patient's activities as he travels through a maze of automated testing procedures. PAs also could be employed to coordinate the clinical care given to patients in multispecialty clinics.

Under a health-team model, PAs could assume roles other than those presently viewed as being within their domain. For instance, instead of functioning in a one-to-one relationship with a physician, they may serve as coordinators and integrators of the entire health care team. Carlson and Athelstan have suggested that electronic information systems for diagnosis, testing, evaluation, and medical record keeping also could fall within the purview of physician's assistants (22). School consultation, industrial medicine, preventive health, and public education are other areas in which PAs could augment their professional duties.

As physician's assistants assume a greater role in coordinating patient care, regulating automated diagnostic services, and supervising other allied health personnel, they will be in a natural position to help us convert from a health-team to a medic-computer model. However, as doctors become obsolete, so too will the physician's assistant. Without any doctors to assist, the concept of a physician's assistant becomes an anachronism. Thus the PA will become a transient figure in medical history. Although he will be an important member of the health care team, the advent of a Post-Physican Era will lead to his eventual demise.

How PAs will define their own professional boundaries, identities, and character in the more immediate future will be interesting to observe. Will their primary loyalties be to the doctors who employ them or to other physician's assistants? Will they decide to run their own training programs rather than be trained under the auspices of the medical profession? Will they unionize? Will they seek to establish their own political hierarchies like nurses and ultimately seek their independence from the medical profession? Will they encourage nurse-practitioners and nurse-clinicians to join their national organizations and to work collectively toward the resolution of common problems? Will nurses be willing to take orders from PAs? The answers to these questions may determine the ultimate character of this new breed of health care professional.

THE PHARMACIST.   While the physician's assistant is striving to find a professional identity, the pharmacist is struggling to recapture his professional dignity. Pharmacy has been described as a profession in search of an occupation. While some believe that the pharmacist is the most overtrained and underutilized member of the health care team, others claim that he is not a member of the team at all. Pharmacy has been referred to as a "marginal profession" in the sense that pharmacists themselves are uncertain if they are primarily professionals or businessmen. One study of pharmacists revealed that if they had it to do all over again, more than half of them would have entered another career (27). Technology coupled with contemporary marketing techniques has led to this disillusionment.

In former times the role of the apothecary was a meaningful one. Equipped with mortar, pestle, and scale, his task was to concoct a heterogeneous collection of seemingly magical elixirs and compounds. He took considerable pride in carefully measuring, mixing, and purifying the remedies he prepared. Over the past 20 to 30 years the art of pharmacy has disappeared as the pharmaceutical industry has turned it into a mass production enterprise (27). Today the pharmacist has been relegated to the role of an entrepreneur whose professional talents have been reduced to counting and dispensing previously manufactured medications. Although he must fill prescriptions with caution and accuracy, he does not need the skills of the apothecary of old. To add insult to injury, the pharmacist is forced to devote more of his time to peddling shampoo than to dispensing drugs. Ironically, as his major responsibilities have become progressively simplified, his education has become increasingly prolonged. He must undergo five years of rigorous training before he is legally sanctioned to count pills. This extensive education has been justified on the grounds that the pharmacist must be cognizant of the biochemistry, metabolism, and clinical effects of medications so that he will be able to inform the doctor of any prescribing errors and to advise his customers about the use of drugs. At this juncture the theoretical expectations and the practical realities of contemporary pharmacy part company.

Because he lacks a knowledge of disease processes, his actual ability to advise customers about medications is severely limited. However, as alleged experts on drugs, some pharmacists hope to maintain their professional dignity by serving as consultants to physicians (28). At least in the immediate future, the pharmacist who seeks professional dignity as a respected consultant may discover his efforts are being ignored by the physician. Although many doctors undoubtedly could benefit from the pharmacist's expertise, most of them will not be willing to take advantage of it. Doctors rarely accept advice from those who are lower in the health care pecking order.

Not only is the pharmacist being ignored by the doctor, but the pharmaceutical industry also is undercutting his authority. Over the years pharmacists have been advocating that physicians prescribe by generic rather than by brand names. In addition to the economic advantages to patients from this policy, the use of generic drug names affords the pharmacist a rare opportunity to exercise professional judgment. For obvious reasons, the pharmaceutical industry opposes the use of generic prescribing and thereby undermines the pharmacist's attempt to maintain whatever minimal professional dignity he still retains (27). Consequently, the contemporary pharmacist serves as an unappreciated intermediary between the medical profession and the pharmaceutical industry. As a result, this highly trained underutilized individual is being left behind to count his pills and type his labels.

Although doctors may be unreceptive to establishing a collaborative relationship with the pharmacist, nurse-practitioners, nurse-clinicians, and physician's assistants may be more willing to do so. If so, the pharmacist may have a greater opportunity to function as a drug consultant under a health-team model. In the more distant future, however, his consultant functions may be usurped by the machine.

Since 1966 the University of Iowa's College of Pharmacy has been running a computerized drug information service for physicians. This automated pharmacopeia informs practitioners about a drug's modes of administration, dosage, side-effects, absorption rates, interactions with other medications, level of toxicity, and so on (29). Other automated systems have been developed that can tell doctors about the effects of drugs upon laboratory test values (30). Computers also have been devised to monitor the prescribing habits of physicians (31–32). Thus, as more automated drug information and monitoring services become available, the consultant functions of the pharmacist may be assumed increasingly by the machine. As a result, the pharmacist will return to dispensing medication.

Although the number of pharmacists and drugstores that will be needed to provide this service is difficult to specify, the American Association of Colleges of Pharmacy has offered some estimates. Their predictions are based upon two major trends. The first is that the number of community pharmacies is declining. In 1900 there were approximately 65,000 community pharmacies; by 1973 the number had fallen to 48,000. The prediction has been made that by 1985 there will be only 40,000 drugstores. The second major trend is that the number of prescriptions will continue to escalate. The number of prescriptions filled in 1972 was 1.4 billion and this number is projected to 3.6 billion by 1985 (33). Another agency, The Futures Group, has forecasted an even greater rise in drug sales. Because new medications will be discovered, drug costs will be covered by national health insurance, and semi-automated dispensing equipment will be available, they predict that the total volume of drug sales in 1970 will be doubled by 1980 and almost tripled by 1985 (34). The simultaneous decrease of community pharmacies and the increasing number of prescriptions will result in fewer drugstores with larger staffs conducting greater volumes of business. In 1972 the typical pharmacy employed 2.2 pharmacists and grossed nearly $120,000 per year. By 1985 it is estimated that the average drugstore will employ 6.8 pharmacists and gross $569,000 annually (1970 dollars) (33). To meet the increasing prescribing habits of physicians and other allied health professionals by 1985 we will need approximately 166,400 additional community pharmacists.

These projections are based upon the assumption that the function of tomorrow's pharmacists will approximate those of today's pharmacist. If his *raison d'être* will be to count pills rather than to advise doctors the need to train ever-increasing numbers of pharmacists has to be questioned. Many hospitals currently train pharmacy technicians or aides in approximately six months to fill prescriptions under the supervision of a licensed pharmacist. In the future the utilization of these technicians could be expanded to reduce the need for highly trained pharmacists.

Conceivably, a "pharmaceutical automat" could be developed in the future. A computer-coded prescription blank could be fed into a machine that would automatically select and count the proper medication. It could label the bottle and maintain a permanent record of the purchase. Computerized financial transactions could be incorporated into the system. Thus, a pharmaceutical automat could relieve the pharmacist of those boring tasks that tend to mechanize him. It also would decrease the need to train additional pharmacists and allow them to devote more of their energies to consultation activities. If the consultation function of the pharmacist will be usurped by a computer and if his counting tasks could be assumed by a pharmaceutical automat, pharmacists eventually may join the physician as a once honored profession that will have outlived its social usefulness.

NEW MEDICAL CAREERS. Although social and technological innovations will render certain health care professions obsolete, these changes also will create new occupations or greatly expand the need for people to enter currently existing ones. For example, I mentioned in Chapter 3 that as the health care system becomes more complex, there will be an increasing demand for medical ombudsmen who will help patients cope with frustrating bureaucracies. The obsolescence of some health care occupations will not entail the obsolescence of all health care occupations. Instead, as historical events evolve, the allocation of medical personnel will change.

Medics. One of the most significant anticipated developments will be the emergence of the medic. His clinical responsibilities have been outlined in the first two chapters of this book. In Chapter 7 I show why it will take only 12 to 18 months for him to be trained. At this point, however, I wish to consider if this brief period of education will enable him to command the respect, and, therefore, the confidence of his patients.

A negative answer to his question would require the acceptance of two dubious assumptions. First, if one respects a practitioner he also will have confidence in him. I have known many patients who have an inordinate respect for their doctor's scientific abilities, but because of their physician's uncaring manner, the patient lacks confidence in him. Although respect is a prerequisite for confidence, respect does not necessarily lead to confidence. Second, a patient's confidence in his clinician does not depend on the healer's education. For centuries shamans and witch doctors commanded the respect and confidence of their clients without having impressive academic credentials. Prevailing cultural or religious ideologies afforded them the prestige that was required to lend credence to their alleged therapeutic powers. Throughout history societies have designated some occupation to fulfill the dependency strivings and omnipotent fantasies of sick individuals. The group that is selected to assume this responsibility derives its authority not only from cultural or religious beliefs, but also from its ability to execute confidence-inspiring rituals. Whereas the shaman would concoct exotic potions, chant mystical incantations, perform in a sanctified setting, and wear ornate costumes, the contemporary physician scrutinizes radiological images, speaks an obscure medical language, practices in a sanitary office, and dresses in a white coat. These activities create a magical aura that not only conforms to prevailing belief systems and enhances the reputation of the clinician, but also has therapeutic benefits for the patient. And finally, in more recent times licensing and certification procedures have legitimized the authority of the practitioner and, thereby, have facilitated his prestige. The essential point, however, is that the attainment of extensive training is not the only way healers acquire the confidence and respect of their patients.

As they have to healers of the past, societies of the future will be able to fashion the medic's role so that he obtains the admiration and trust of his patients. The process by which society accomplishes this objective has never been and never will be systematically, deliberately, or consciously planned. Instead, it will flow naturally and inconspicuously from the prevailing norms, values, practices, and expectations of the culture. Although medics will not have a lengthy education, they will still have some specialized accredited training. Like the shaman and physician who preceded him, the medic will perform rituals, such as utilizing complicated machines, practicing in uniquely designed settings, conversing in a strange clinical vocabulary, and wearing a futuristic medical uniform. Furthermore, licensing and certification procedures will enhance his prestige. Thus, the medic's authority will be fostered by the clinical rituals and accouterments of a Post-Physician Era.

There are other reasons why medics will be able to command the respect and confidence of their patients. When contrasting the extensively trained doctor of today with the lesser trained medic of tomorrow, naturally the medic would not appear capable of receiving our admiration and trust. Nevertheless, in the future this comparison will become meaningless. In a Post-Physician Era medics will be the primary health care practitioners. If comparisons will be made, they will not be between the medic and the doctor but rather between the new medic-computer model and the old physician-centered or health-team model.

My experience with mental health workers leads me to believe that confidence and respect in one's therapist is more a product of the personality and sensitivity of the clinician than it is a function of his academic credentials. Although many patients initially prefer to see a doctor, once a therapeutic alliance has been established, formal degrees and titles exert an inconsequential or minimal effect upon ultimate treatment results.* Because the medic's primary task will be supportive rather than technical, I believe that he will be able to command the respect and confidence of his patients, just as many contemporary mental health workers are respected by their own clients.

Medical Computer and Communication Technologists. As the machine assumes an expanded medical role, the computer expert will become a vital member of the health care team. An automated medical system would grind to a halt without him. It would be unreasonable, if not undesirable, to expect that doctors, PAs, nurse-clinicians, and others will learn the technical intricacies of the computer. Not only would this task detract them from expanding their clinical knowledge and from attending their patients, but they are probably not suited by temperament to do so. Because a medic-computer model is so dependent on the machine, computer technologists would have to be available within a medical facility on an around-the-clock basis. They would have to correct minor technical problems, and ensure that backup systems are ready to function in case primary automated decision-making apparati fail to operate. Furthermore, some hospitals have been temporarily stymied in their initial use of computers because they have not had an adequate number of these experts (15, 35–36). The introduction of automated techniques as well as the eventual actualization of a Post-Physician Era, will be contingent upon the existence of computer technologists.

Many technical and psychological factors must be considered if medical computer specialists are to maximize their effectiveness.

---

* I must emphasize that this assertion is only my impression. Adequate studies to confirm or refute this hypothesis have yet to be performed.

They will need to be familiar with the problems of designing medical computer programs and implementing them within a clinical setting. They also will need to be aware of the emotional reactions of health care professionals to the computer. Whereas many businessmen view the machine as a profitable time-saving device, many doctors view the computer as a threat to their omnipotence and independence. Computer specialists need to be sensitive to these concerns and to devise helpful and supportive ways of responding to them. Medical computer specialists could advantageously spend part of their training within medical and nursing schools. They could have sessions with student-physicians and nurses wherein the problems of using computers within a medical setting and their psychological reactions to doing so could be freely aired. Practicing nurses and doctors could hold similar meetings. In whatever way the dialog between health care personnel and computer specialists is established, the critical points are that such a dialog needs to exist and that medical computer specialists must familiarize themselves with the unique technical and emotional problems of working in hospitals and clinics. Training computer experts to work in a medical context is different from preparing them to work in other settings.

Much of what has been mentioned in regard to computer specialists also applies to communication technologists. As the use of sophisticated communication systems in the delivery of medical services expands, the demand for these specialists will increase. Communication technologists have to consider the unique requirements of working within medical institutions. For example, using television cameras for public entertainment presents problems that are different from using them for health care delivery. Cameramen must be sensitive to the needs of patients (e.g., they should not be intrusive), and they must distinguish what is clinically important from what is medically irrelevant. They also will have to place health considerations (e.g., maintaining sterile operating room conditions) above technical requirements (e.g., placing of cameras, lights, and sound equipment). To become aware of these factors communication technologists should receive a portion of their training within a medical setting.

Undoubtedly, computer and communication experts will play a greater role in the future of medicine. Nevertheless, there are serious questions if medical professionals will be receptive to their efforts and include them as full-fledged members of the health care team. Studying how these emerging professional groups can become integral members of the health care team represents only one focus of investigation for future medical researchers.

THE MEDICAL RESEARCHER.   Medical researchers include a wide diversity of investigators whose ultimate mission is to improve man's health. These scientists come not only from medicine, but from other disciplines, such as biology, psychology, chemistry, physics, economics, engineering, administration, mathematics, and sociology. Although the lay public usually gives physicians the credit for discovering medical breakthroughs, other professions have played an equally important role in the advancement of medical knowledge. To specify which group of medical researchers has rendered the most significant contributions would be absurd, because each discipline is dependent upon the findings of the other to make their discoveries. Although this interdependence is generally recognized, all too often this awareness is not fully translated into organizational terms. This unfortunate reality is more apparent in universities, where frequently each discipline maintains its own rigid boundaries. Often one finds the ludicrous situation in which psychologists do not talk to psychiatrists, who do not talk to surgeons, who do not talk to microbiologists, who do not talk to ecologists, and so on. Institutional barriers inhibit the cross-fertilization of ideas and, therefore, retard the growth of medical knowledge. Academicians recognize the importance of interdisciplinary projects, but are painfully aware of the frustrations that often accompany attempts to sustain interdepartmental programs.

I do not wish to convey the notion that interdisciplinary investigations do not occur; I only want to emphasize that if future medical researchers are to maximize their productivity, new organizational structures may need to be devised. One way of doing so would be through the establishment of Schools of Medical Investigation, a topic to be discussed further in Chapter 7. For now, however, I wish to note that if interdisciplinary research is to be fostered, it may require more than the admirable intentions of scientists. Private and government funding may have to be channeled into the development of institutions, such as Schools of Medical Investigation, to maximize collaborative research.

Undoubtedly, by enhancing the collection of factual data, computers and other forms of technological instrumentation will accelerate the pace of future medical research. But to overemphasize the importance of these technical aids would be a mistake. Heightened imagination, intuition, and perceptivity will advance medical knowledge more than the simple accumulation and manipulation of facts. As F. M. Berger has observed, "While knowledge of all relevant facts is a prerequisite for making a discovery, discovery is more than knowing all the facts" (37, p. 69). For example, although many scientists had previously noted that penicillium mold inhibited the growth of bacteria, it took Fleming's thoughtful observation and special imagination to recognize the ultimate significance of this phenomenon. Regardless of how sophisticated, no computer could have discovered penicillin. Although technological and social change may render many of the health care professions obsolete, medical researchers will not undergo a similar fate. Technology will provide researchers with new methods for investigating old problems; areas that formerly were unexplorable by conventional techniques will be accessible as innovative methods become available. Consequently, technology not only will facilitate the work of the medical researcher, but it also will afford him a greater number of topics to study (38).

In recent years there has been a tendency to denigrate the value of scientific investigations. Since 1967 the federal government has curtailed financial support of medical research (39). The widespread skepticism toward scientists and their work has been partially responsible for this trend. I discuss this problem as well as some of the more controversial areas of future medical research in the following chapter. At this juncture, however, I want to emphasize that medical professionals, politicians, and the public need to take a closer look at what scientists ought to be investigating. Given our limited fiscal resources, research priorities that ultimately will provide the greatest good for the greatest number must be established. What is topical is not always relevant, and what is relevant is not always apparent. Therefore, where should we place our research priorities?

Franz Ingelfinger has made a useful distinction between what he calls the "have" and the "have-not" diseases. The former are those fatal conditions, such as heart disease, stroke, and cancer, that are the most intense objects of scientific investigation; enormous amounts of money are spent to find a remedy for them. "Have-not" diseases are cripplers, rather than killers, and include illnesses such as emphysema, arthritis, asthma, and ulcerative colitis. Although these latter disorders may affect a larger proportion of the populace than the "have" diseases, funds to discover a cure for them are in relatively short supply (40). Moreover, killer diseases remove the patient as a consumer shortly after he stops being a producer, whereas crippling disorders leave the patient as a consumer long after he ceases being a' producer. To be afflicted by a "have-not" disease is depressing to the individual and wasteful to his family and society. Sometimes even death itself is preferable. Because to live in a certain way is more important than to die in a certain way, allocating a greater portion of our limited research funds to the understanding and cure of the "have-not" diseases might be better than to succumb to politicians and special health lobbies who capitalize upon the public's preoccupation with the "have" illnesses (40). As the life span of our populace increases, the crippling diseases will affect a relatively greater number of people. It is of dubious value to save these individuals from killer diseases, if they are to be subjected to the immobilizing infirmities that often accompany prolonged life (41). We should attempt to encourage public officials to spend a proportionately larger amount of the medical research dollar on the "have-not" disorders.

To help us choose worthwhile research priorities, Lewis Thomas has distinguished between the "High Technology" and the "Halfway Technology" of medicine. The former derives from a basic understanding of disease mechanisms, is highly effective in curing illness, and is relatively inexpensive and easy to deliver. Examples of this High Technology include immunizations against diphtheria and polio, antibiotics for the treatment of pneumonia, tuberculosis, and syphilis, hormones for the correction of endocrine dysfunctions, and nutritional therapy for preventing the manifestations of certain inherited and acquired disorders. The Halfway Technology of medicine refers to treatment interventions that compensate for the disabling effects of some illnesses without substantially altering their ultimate course. Their purpose is to palliate symptoms and to postpone death rather than curing disease. Examples of treatment methods derived from Halfway Technology are renal dialysis and organ transplantation. These forms of therapy are usually difficult and costly to deliver, relatively painful and frequently dangerous to the patient, and have a variable degree of effectiveness. Despite the advantages of treatments derived from High Technology, generally the measures resulting from Halfway Technology capture the public's attention. The inordinate publicity afforded heart transplantation illustrates what Thomas means when he observes, "The media tend to present each new (Halfway Technology) procedures as though it represented a breakthrough and therapeutic triumph, instead of the makeshift that it really is" (39, p. 31).

Because the products of Halfway Technology research look spectacular, receive a "good press," and appear effective, it has been tempting to support these endeavors. Because High Technology research often involves basic laboratory investigation, is complicated for laymen to understand, and usually does not appear to have practical value, or to immediately yield dramatic results, it tends to be labeled as "irrelevant." As a result, Thomas correctly argues that professionals, politicians, and the public have mistakenly favored Halfway Technology research. In terms of both money and human suffering, the costs of deploying iron lungs to thousands of polio victims are overwhelming in comparison to offering mass polio inoculations. Similarly, if today one used the best Halfway Technology for treating typhoid fever that was available in 1935, the patient would have to remain in the hospital for about 50 days, receive methodical nursing care, require extensive laboratory tests, need occasional emergency abdominal surgery, and pay at least $10,000. Furthermore, there would be a good chance that the patient would not even survive. High Technology research has provided us with chloramphenicol that can treat typhoid fever relatively quickly, inexpensively, and effectively (39). Thomas uses these illustrations to support his contention that High Technology medicine should be our top research priority rather than the stopgap measures that accrue from Halfway Technology investigations.

Underlying his argument is the belief that medicine must engage in technological assessment just as other industries do. We must know if we are getting the maximum benefit from our research dollars. I concur with Thomas' conviction that this can best be accomplished by favoring and supporting High Technology research, even though this approach lacks popular appeal. If this priority is to prevail, however, and if future generations of medical investigators are to receive the financial assistance they will deserve, they will have to educate both funding agencies and the public to the importance of High Technology research; they might even have to convince themselves of this fact.

Although many individuals may dispute the priorities I have suggested, if worthwhile medical research is to flourish, investigators will need to justify not only the medical and economic merits of their work, but also the ethical consequences that may arise from it. Biomedical research is already under attack for delving into areas that may alter the fundamental nature of our species. Expected discoveries in aging, genetic manipulation, reproduction, behavioral control, and organ transplantation may increase the intensity of these assaults. Discussions of these topics are sometimes so emotionally charged that sense and nonsense become confused. If we are to avoid this pitfall and to avert a backlash against medical research, we must soberly place these issues within their proper scientific and ethical perspectives.

NOTES

1. B. S. Eisenberg, and P. Aherne (eds.) (1974). *Socioeconomic Issues of Health '74.* Chicago: American Medical Association.

2. Erikson, E. H. (1968). *Identity: Youth and Crisis.* New York: Norton.

3. Sadler, A. M., Jr., B. L. Sadler, and A. A. Bliss (1972). *The Physician's Assistant: Today and Tomorrow.* New Haven: Yale University Press.

4. Altman, S. H. (1972). *Present & Future Supply of Registered Nurses.* Bethesda, Md.: U.S. Department of Health, Education, and Welfare. DHEW Publication Number (NIH) 73-134.

5. Bates, B. (1970). "Doctor and Nurse: Changing Roles and Relations." *New England Journal of Medicine,* 283:129-134.

6. Rockoff, M. A. (1973). "Interactions Between Medical Students and Nursing Personnel." *Journal of Medical Education,* 48:725-731.

7. *American Medical News* (1970). "Health Manpower Shortages," 13(30):6.

8. Field, M. G. (1973). "The Concept of the 'Health System' at the Macro-Sociological Level." Mimeo.

9. Paynich, M. L. (1971). "Why Do Basic Nursing Students Work in Nursing?" *Nursing Outlook,* 19:242-245.

10. National Commission for the Study of Nursing and Nursing Education (1970). *An Abstract for Action.* New York: McGraw-Hill.

11. Freidson, E. (1972). *Profession of Medicine: A Study of the Sociology of Applied Knowledge.* New York: Dodd, Mead.

12. Silver, H. K., and P. A. McAtee (1972). "Who Will Provide More Health Care?—II" *Medical Tribune,* 13(48):5.

13. Holleran, C. (1972). "The Now Nurse." *Medical Opinion and Review,* 7(1): 20-26.

14. Rutstein, D. D. (1967). *The Coming Revolution in Medicine.* Cambridge, Mass.: M.I.T. Press.

15. *Computers and Medicine* (1974). " 'Vital'— A Real Time Hospital Information System," 3(4):1-2.

16. Kadish, J., and J. W. Long (1970). "The Training of Physician Assistants: Status and Issues." *Journal of the American Medical Association,* 212:1047-1051.

17. Hudson, C. L. (1961). "Physicians Assistant: Expansion of Medical Professional Services with Nonprofessional Personnel." *Journal of the American Medical Association,* 176:839-841.

18. Fisher, D. W. (1974). Personal Communication, October 24.

19. Hendrickson, R. M. (1974). "Solo Vs. Group Practice." *Prism,* 2(11):28-29.

20. *Medical World News* (1973). "After Eight Years: Duke's PA Program," 14(19):68.

21. Department of Health Manpower Division of Medical Practice (N.D.). *Employment & Use of Physician's Assistants: A Guide for Physicians.* Chicago: American Medical Association.

22. Carlson, C. L., and G. T. Athelstan (1970). "The Physician's Assistant: Versions and Diversions of A Promising Concept." *Journal of the American Medical Association,* 214:1855–1861.

23. Light, I. (1969). "Development and Growth of New Allied Health Fields." *Journal of the American Medical Association,* 210:114–120.

24. Lohrenz, F. N. (1971). "The Marshfield Clinic Physician-Assistant Concept." *New England Journal of Medicine,* 284:301–304.

25. Todd, M. C., and D. F. Foy (1972). "Current Status of the Physician's Assistant and Related Issues." *Journal of the American Medical Association,* 220:1714–1720.

26. National Academy of Sciences (1970). *New Members of the Physician's Health Team: Physician's Assistants.* Report of the Ad Hoc Panel on New Members of the Physician's Health Team of the Board on Medicine of the National Academy of Sciences. Washington, D.C.

27. Smith, M. C. (1974). "Can You Dispense with Pharmacists?" *Medical Marketing and Media,* 9(6):28–31.

28. Csáky, T. Z. (1973). "Clinical Pharmacy and Pharmacology: Friends or Foes?" *Journal of Medical Education,* 48:905–910.

29. *Medical World News* (1973). "Drug Index Supplies Latest Data," 14(15):31.

30. *Medical World News* (1973). "Computerizing Drugs' Effect on Tests," 14 (18):71.

31. Wade, O. L. (1968). "The Computer and Drug Prescribing." In G. McLachlan, and R. A. Shegog (eds.), *Computers in the Service of Medicine: Essays on Current Research and Applications, Volume I.* London: Oxford University Press. Pp. 151–162.

32. *Computers and Medicine* (1974). "An Ambulatory Care Information System (Continued)," 3(6):3.

33. Rodowskas, C. A., Jr. (1973). "Pharmacy Manpower: Current Status and Future Requirements." *Medical Marketing and Media,* 8(7):18–30.

34. *The Futurist* (1974). "Pharmaceutical Sales to Double by 1980," 8:247.

35. Sidel, V. W. (1971). "New Technologies and the Practice of Medicine." In E. Mendelsohn, J. P. Swazey, and I. Taviss (eds.), *Human Aspects of Biomedical Innovation.* Cambridge: Harvard University Press. Pp. 131–155.

36. *Computers and Medicine* (1973). "MIS-1 After A Full Year's Operation—Pros & Cons," 2(6):1, 2, & 4.

37. Berger, F. M. (1967). "Computers and Medical Discoveries." *Perspectives in Biology and Medicine,* 11:63–70.

38. Handler, P. (ed.) (1970). *Biology and the Future of Man.* New York: Oxford University Press.

39. Thomas, L. (1974). "The Future Impact of Science and Technology on Medicine." *Bulletin of the American College of Surgeons,* 59(6):25–35.

40. Ingelfinger, F. J. (1972). "Haves and Have-Nots in the World of Disease." *New England Journal of Medicine,* **287**:1198–1199.

41. Ehrlich, G. E. (1973). "Health Challenges of the Future." *The Annals of the American Academy of Political and Social Science,* **408**:70–82.

6

DRACONIAN IMAGES
AND THE
NEW BIOLOGY_____

"Contemporary Americans are accustomed to seeing science fiction become scientific fact" (1, p. 1). If true, this observation provides a clue as to why the anticipated biomedical revolution has intrigued and frightened mankind. Although third-rate horror films can be readily dismissed as amusing diversions, their popularity may also reflect a cultural attitude of considerable importance to medicine's future. Typically, these movies portray a mad doctor who transgresses the laws of man and God by creating and unleashing the ultimate monster. As the agent of the evil physician's alter ego, the creature terrorizes the simple village folk and attacks the lovely heroine. In the end, however, virtue triumphs. In the nick of time the fair maiden is rescued by her God-fearing scientist-beau. The sinister doctor is murdered by the fiend, who is then destroyed by the enraged citizenry under the inspired leadership of the youthful scientist. The moral is always the same. Divine wisdom has ordained that a total understanding of the biological secrets of life must never be acquired by man. If one fails to respect this taboo, cataclysmic consequences are inevitable. As a latter-day Adam, the brilliant doctor's pathologic lust for knowledge seduces him to partake of the forbidden fruit. The resultant catastrophe serves as a warning to future generations that man's curiosity must be circumscribed if salvation is to be realized. It is not science *per se*, but rather the abuses of science that generate evil. As long as the scientist does not tamper with the mysteries of creation, he shall receive the Almighty's blessing and protection.

These themes are not limited to the screen. What had been merely religious faith or cinemagraphic fantasy has now become scientific reality. The prospect of a biomedical revolution has resurrected the fear that man is intruding upon knowledge that only God should possess. Alarmists exclaim:

> You may not know it, but you are living in the middle of the biological revolution—and its time bomb is ticking remorselessly for you, for all of us. . . . Within a very few years, the world around us will be changed beyond recognition. There will be no sex, no death, no human body—as we know them. We may see people buying chastity or desire at a drug store, groups of absolutely identical people—supermen, geniuses or perhaps monsters, the manufacture of half-men-half-machines, a pill to stop—or start—human aggression, the total destruction of human "identity" (2, p. i).

We are entering upon a revolutionary period in biological medicine. Projected discoveries in reproduction, genetic engineering, organ modification, aging, and behavioral control will force man to reexamine his ethical standards, legal systems, evolutionary alternatives, and most of all, his definition of self. These issues demand attention. Nevertheless, to become mesmerized by the dire caveats of those who predict that the new biology will plunge mankind into a Draconian world order is absurd, if not dangerous. Unrestrained hysteria, sensationalism, and threats will only encumber our efforts to cope with the biomedical revolution. Later in this chapter some of the pitfalls and opportunities for contending with the consequences of future biomedical innovations are discussed. First, however, a brief survey of some of these developments and their implications are explored.

THE NEW BIOLOGY.   For many of us high school biology dealt with nondescript plants and hideous insects. Unlike this "old" biology, the new biology is highly relevant to man, and it has captured his imagination. Countless articles and books have been written, explicating the scientific, ethical, social, legal, and psychological consequences of the new biology. To provide a comprehensive review of this multifaceted subject would be impossible within a single chapter, but a brief summary of the topic may help to familiarize the unacquainted with some of its more critical dimensions.

Organ Replacement. The subject of organ replacement exemplifies the dictum "the future is now." Although still a highly experimental procedure, within a decade heart transplantation may become as routine as kidney transplantation is today. In the future everything from lungs to limbs may be transplanted (2–3), especially if the problems of immunologic rejection are solved. This latter difficulty is not insurmountable. Rejection problems may be overcome in three principal ways: minimizing the differences between the antigens of the donor and those of the recipient, administering immuno-suppressive drugs, and inducing specific tolerance of the foreign transplantation agents. Even today, by using a combination of these techniques, 80 percent of kidney grafts can function adequately for at least two years (4).

From a strictly surgical perspective, the optimal source of a transplant is from another *living human subject*. This is so because the donor organ is in a relatively healthy state and can be transferred at the patient's, donor's, and physician's convenience. When the graft is a paired organ, such as a kidney, a living donor is usually a viable possibility. However, when the graft is a nonpaired organ, such as a heart, alternative contributors must be found. In these circumstances the surgeon must rely upon organs from *recently deceased patients*. The use of cadaveric specimens presents both immunologic and storage problems. Storing potentially transplantable organs entails a great deal more than simply placing them in a refrigerator. Prolonged freezing can damage tissues by forming ice crystals and by concentrating salts (2). Therefore, at least at present, cadaveric specimens must be implanted soon after the donor has expired. In the future, however, if storage problems can be overcome, organ banks may be widely established in which tissues are typed and relevant data about potential donors and recipients are entered into a computer (5). Such banks exist for blood, skin, bone, and corneas. *Living animals* are a third presently available, albeit infrequently utilized, donor source. Although the immunologic problems are greater than those of living human grafts, animal tissues would have the advantage of relieving surgeons of the burden of finding human contributors.

The transplantation of organs has generated a myriad of significant questions. What constitutes free and informed consent? Are children fully able to comprehend the consequences of donating an organ? Are prisoners, desperately hoping for a parole, truly free to give their consent? What about the reluctant donor who is subtly coerced by social or family pressure to contribute one of his organs? Hopefully, an alert physician might detect this pressure and state that the donor is medically unsuitable, thereby protecting him from social ostracism and personal guilt (6).

Other problems emerge when a transplanted organ comes from an individual who has recently died. One major dilemma is to determine if the potential donor is actually deceased. Death is not a temporally circumscribed event; man and his parts die in degrees (7). Moreover, because modern resuscitative techniques can perpetuate cardiac activity long after the brain has ceased to function,* physicians have had to reexamine their definition of

---

* This fact has led Dr. Willard Gaylin to propose the establishment of "bio-emporiums" where recently brain dead cadavers or "neomorts" would be stored with their noncerebral physiologic functions being maintained. These neomorts could be used to train physicians; to test drugs and surgical pro-

death (9). Although the termination of neurological instead of cardiovascular activity is gradually becoming the accepted criterion for death (10), no medical or legal consensus on this issue exists. Until this occurs, doctors risk a malpractice suit when utilizing an organ from an apparently deceased individual (7). An overzealous surgeon, preoccupied with saving his patient's life, may prematurely extract an organ from a potentially savable victim. To a large extent this pitfall can be obviated by having the determination of death rendered by a physician other than the one seeking to perform the transplant (11).

Another difficult issue is determining who should receive a transplanted organ. Scarce medical and financial resources necessitate that choices be made. Although "medical need" rather than "social worth" has allegedly been the criterion for making these decisions (1), a discrepancy exists between theory and practice. For example, among the first 100 American heart transplants there were 64 black donors and only one black recipient (12). Although this fact may reveal more about American society than it does about transplantation surgery, it reminds us that the practice of medicine is not immune from cultural prejudices.

In the future three other donor sources may be used. One possibility would be to develop organs from *embryonic tissue*, while another would be to grow duplicate organs from healthy cells derived from the patient's own *defective organ*. Because of technical difficulties, the utilization of both of these sources may not be possible for another 50 to 100 years. However, the use of *artificial organs* may have a more immediate impact. Because the heart has a relatively simple structure, it probably will be the first major artificial implantable organ to be utilized—techniques for implanting bone, teeth, and arteries already exist (3). Within a decade a totally implantable artificial heart may be ready for clinical use (1, 13), but before this is accomplished, the problems of immunologic rejection, material reliability, blood

cedures; to store potentially transplantable organs; and to serve as continuing sources for blood, bone marrow, skin, corneas, cartilage, hormones, antibodies, antitoxins, and so on (8).

clotting, and adequate power supplies must be resolved (2, 5, 14).

Originally, prostheses were intended merely to substitute for diseased organs in otherwise healthy individuals. Their use in preventing death could prolong life. Some believe that their use in counteracting the effects of aging would be unlikely, because the aging process is a gradual deterioration of tissues in which certain organs degenerate before others. Therefore, the implantation of artificial organs in elderly individuals would be a perpetual necessity. However, patients may be unlikely to refuse a prosthesis just because another organ will become dysfunctional within several years (2). If so, the demand for artificial organs could escalate.

Despite nature's ingenious artistry, artificial devices may improve upon the human product, and eventually people may replace their organs freely. If so, humanity would enter a new stage of history in which the semiartificial man becomes a reality. Man and machine could be intermeshed so completely that the two would become indistinguishable. This hybrid, known as a "cyborg" (an abbreviation for cybernetic organism), would be capable of two-way communication between its human and mechanical parts. Computers and other sophisticated devices could be implanted in man to amplify his intellectual or physical powers (2). The potential implications are mind-boggling. Pessimists fear that conflicts between men and cyborgs could lead to nothing less than a total annihilation of human culture. Conversely, optimists proclaim that eventually natural selection will allow cyborgs to dominate and enrich civilization (15). Regardless of one's point of view the mechanization of humans and the humanization of machines could have profound consequences (16).

Reproduction. Our expanding knowledge of the reproductive process will produce a wide array of clinical techniques and social dilemmas. Before I describe some of these, a brief outline of normal human reproductive physiology might be useful.

Under the influence of gonadotropic hormones, the ovaries

release an egg into the oviduct. There it is fertilized by a spermatozoa and becomes an embryo. By a process known as "cleavage,"
the embryo divides into two equal cells, then four, eight, and so
on. During this time it travels down the oviduct; when it consists
of approximately 16 cells, it enters the uterus. The embryo
continues to divide until it becomes a blastocyst, a 64-celled
structure enveloping a fluid-filled cavity. The blastocyst implants
onto the uterine wall and develops rapidly into a recognizable
fetus.

Although incompletely understood, this entire process is
regulated by hormones. It is not surprising, therefore, that
developments in endocrinology are being applied to alter normal
reproductive functions. The most well-known use of hormones
has been with birth control pills, which generally inhibit the
release of eggs from the ovaries. In the near future other
hormonal agents will be available, such as night-before and
morning-after pills, long-acting injections, implantable time-
release capsules, and male contraceptives (17). Eventually, the
use of contraceptives in public water supplies may provide a
vehicle for massive population control. A special antidote would
have to be administered to a woman to allow her to have a child
(16). Whether this program would be technically feasible or
ethically desirable remains to be seen. Although the use of
hormones generally has been associated with birth control, they
also can be utilized to facilitate pregnancy and to heighten sexual
desire. As Gordon Taylor has stated, "We are moving out of the
phase of crude 'birth-control' into a new era for which the term
'fertility-control' seems more appropriate" (2, pp. 49–50).

Another way to enhance fertility, especially for couples who
cannot have children because the husband's sperm are inadequate,
is by artificial insemination with donor (AID). With this procedure, sperm (usually from an anonymous contributor) are
mechanically introduced into the uterus. Although AID has been
used to conceive more than 150,000 Americans during the past 15
years (2), the law does not clearly define the rights of the offspring. As of 1974, in all but two states (Oklahoma and Georgia),
children derived from AID are considered illegitimate, even

though the father and mother approve of the procedure (18). Because of the potentially damaging financial and psychological consequences of being labeled illegitimate, a rectification of existing legal codes seems justified (17–18).

More complicated ethical and legal problems may arise when another technique, artificial inovulation (AI) is widely performed in humans. With this procedure, fertilized eggs are extracted from the oviduct or the uterus of one animal and implanted into the womb of another. This technique can result in a white rabbit giving birth to a black rabbit, or a Friesian cow producing a Hereford calf. Furthermore, when gonadatropic hormones are injected into a donor animal, its ovaries are stimulated to release a greater number of eggs. These eggs can be fertilized and allowed to develop in other uteri. In this way a greater number of offspring from prized animals can be produced. Artificial inovulation could help women whose oviducts are blocked so that their eggs are unable to reach the uterus. In the future the greater application of AI in humans will generate a wide array of controversial issues. For example, would the donor or the recipient be the child's biological or legal mother? What would be the psychosocial consequences of a white mother giving birth to a black child or vice versa? These questions would not arise if the egg is implanted in the donor's uterus, but by "renting" another's womb, some women will be able to have their "own" children without having to undergo a pregnancy. A new occupation, the "professional breeder," could emerge. Whereas some may view this development as a further stage in the emancipation of women, others may see it as a desecration of motherhood.

Similar beliefs may be held about the artificial placenta. It works by having the fetal umbilical cord pass through a lightly coiled cellulose tube where it is bathed in an oxygen-enriched fluid. Already this machine has kept a 26-week old human fetus alive for five hours (2). Although many complex technical problems remain, eventually the artificial placenta could play a useful clinical role. It could provide an alternative to abortion for mothers whose lives are threatened by a pregnancy. Theoretically, the fetus could be transferred from her uterus to an artificial placenta, thereby saving the life of both mother and child. The impact of the mechanical womb upon society may cause some people to fear the emergence of a Brave New World; others will look forward to having the joys of motherhood without the discomforts of pregnancy. Conceivably, an artificial placenta that would outperform the natural one could be fabricated. If so, some women actually may prefer the mechanical womb. However, by continuing to develop this machine an ethical question has been raised. Paul Ramsey observes:

> The decisive moral verdict must be that we cannot rightfully *get to know* how to do this without conducting unethical experiments upon the unborn who must be the "mishaps" (the dead and the retarded ones) through whom we learn how. It is amazing that, in discussions of man's self-modification of the future of his species by prenatal refabrication, this simple, decisive ethical objection is so seldom mentioned. This can only mean that our ethos is well prepared to make human waste for the sake of these self-elected goals (19, pp. 113–114). (Ramsey's italics).

This objection cannot be readily dismissed; it applies not only to the invention of the artificial placenta, but also to *any* experiments that attempt to modify prenatal development. *

One such example would be in the use of *in vitro* fertilization. Although the technical details have not been worked out, essentially it entails obtaining an egg from a women's ovaries and fertilizing it with a man's spermatozoa in a laboratory. R. G. Edwards, a pioneer in this field, has been able to grow impregnated eggs to the blastocyst stage (20).

Dr. Pyotr Anakhin of the Academy of Medical Science in Moscow has claimed that his team maintained 250 embryos for considerably longer periods of time. In one case the embryo survived six months and weighed $1\frac{1}{2}$ pounds (17). By implanting these embryos into a uterus, *in vitro* fertilization will allow previously infertile couples to have children. It could help women with occluded oviducts and men who have developed antibodies to

---

* Later in this chapter the general ethical issues of prenatal and developmental experimentation are discussed more extensively.

their own spermatozoa or who have inadequate sperm counts. In the more distant future this technique may benefit couples with a high risk of having a child with a serious genetic illness. For example, diseases such as hemophilia usually afflict only males. Because eventually it will be possible to determine the sex of an *in vitro* fertilized blastocyst, only female embryos could be implanted in women who fear that they will have a defective offspring (20).

Recognizing that normal pregnancy also entails risks, Marc Lappé has justified couples consenting to this procedure if they are fully apprised of the known dangers of the technique and cannot get help by any other method (21). Paul Ramsey objects to the use of *in vitro* fertilization because in developing it, a seriously impaired child may be inadvertently created. He argues that to rationalize this potential danger on the basis that normal pregnancy also involves risks is like saying that one mistake justifies another (19). However, if one takes Ramsey's argument to its logical extreme, all experimentation would be unethical. Since every medical development was at one time in the experimental stage, the adoption of Ramsey's position would have made the practice of medicine itself unethical.

The availability of sperm and egg banks will facilitate the widespread use of AID, AI, and *in vitro* fertilization. Spermatozoa frozen in liquid nitrogen have retained their potency for more than 10 years. Moreover, in a documented series of 400 births using frozen semen, no increase in abnormalities has been apparent. Currently, sperm banks have been established in England, Japan, and in 20 American cities. Although costs vary, one Baltimore firm charges $80 for the initial collection and an annual storage fee of $18 (22). One immediate reason for the growth of sperm banks has been the increased popularity of vasectomies. Surgeons usually are not able to reverse a vasectomy; so, by storing their sperm, vasectomized men will be able to have children at some future date (23). Another current use of frozen semen is for men with inadequate sperm counts. Spermatazoa from numerous ejaculations can be collected, concentrated, frozen, and eventually inseminated artificially. Some authors have suggested that frozen sperm, which are protected from radio-activity, might be valuable in the aftermath of a nuclear holocaust (2, 17). Eugenicists believe that in the more distant future sperm from "exceptional" people could be stored, and thereby used to improve humanity's gene pool.

Although considerable progress in freezing spermatozoa has been made, similar advancements with eggs have yet to be accomplished. However, the establishment of ovum as well as blastocyst banks appears inevitable (17).

All of the techniques that have been mentioned involve sexual reproduction—that is, a process by which fetal development occurs after a union of a sperm and an egg. Within the next 50 years man may be able to replicate his species by a form of asexual reproduction known as "cloning." This technique was developed by English zoologist John Gurdon who performed the following experiment. By means of radiation he destroyed the haploid nucleus of a frog egg and replaced it with a diploid nucleus * derived from a frog's intestinal cell. Several months later his specimen developed into an exact replicate of the donor frog. Under normal circumstances genetic material comes from both parents; this animal's chromosomes were derived exclusively from the donor frog. Because its genetic material came from a somatic cell, it contained the full number of chromosomes. By cloning, the creation of two, 200, or even 2,000 *genetically* identical animals is theoretically possible.

In the future the same could be done with man. This does not mean, however, that people cloned from the same cell would be exact replicates of one another. One-egg (monozygotic), or so-called "identical twins," are identical only in their genetic makeup. Their behavior, personality, intelligence, appearance, and even their biological state may differ enormously depending upon how the environment has altered the expression of their

---

* The chromosomes of all cells are located within the nucleus. Eggs and sperm (i.e., the sex cells) are considered to be haploid—that is, they contain half the adult number of chromosomes. Every other cell in the body (i.e., the somatic cells) are considered to be diploid—that is, they possess the full complement of chromosomes.

genetic material. If one member of a monozygotic pair is nurtured by stimulating and caring parents, exercises frequently, eats properly, and does not contract a serious illness, he may grow up to be an intelligent, charming, muscular, and healthy adult. If the other twin is raised by dull and insensitive people, exercises rarely, eats poorly, and has tuberculosis, he may grow up to be a stupid, obnoxious, scrawny, and sickly individual. Because people are the product of genetic and environmental interactions, monozygotic twins or clonants with the same hereditary constitution could become markedly different individuals. Therefore, to say that cloning could automatically and simply produce 47 Mozarts or 147 Hitlers is absurd. Accomplishing this feat would necessitate the existence of not only identical genetic makeups, but also of identical environmental experiences. Although the relative importance that heredity and environment ultimately play in determining an individual's behavior, personality, intelligence, appearance, and biology are still controversial, clearly both factors make significant contributions.

Cloned persons could receive transplanted organs without fear of immunologic rejection. Therefore, in the future everyone may wish to be cloned in the event that someday they will require a transplant. Moreover, those carrying healthy genes may prefer to clone themselves, rather than to risk producing defective children by sexual reproduction.

The major advantage of cloning would be to perpetuate individuals with desirable genetic qualities. However, deciding upon what qualities are desirable and who should be cloned present difficult problems. To the extent that genetics do influence a person's characteristics, would we, for example, wish to clone a Fidel Castro? The answer may rest upon what we think about Fidel Castro. Furthermore, whose opinion should prevail? Should the decision be left to scientists and politicians? Should anybody be allowed to clone themselves?

Eugenists hope that the quality of the gene pool will be improved by cloning healthy individuals. However, even the proponents of cloning admit that an *exclusive* reliance upon this technique would be an inadvisable way of perpetuating the species.

Those who are cloned from exceptional individuals would have a considerable survival advantage, but in the long run because of their fixed genetic makeup, clonants may be unable to adapt satisfactorily to environmental change. A species composed entirely of cloned men eventually would become extinct in an evolutionary cul-de-sac. Consequently, some experts have suggested that society use both forms of reproduction—sexual reproduction for heterogeneity and innovation and asexual reproduction for uniformity and multiplying proven excellence. As, Joshua Lederberg has recommended, "A mix of sexual and clonal reproduction makes good sense for genetic design. Leave sexual reproduction for experimental purposes; when a suitable type is ascertained take care to maintain it by clonal propagation" (19, p. 73).

What Lederberg feels is genetically desirable, Ramsey believes is ethically offensive. He recoils at the thought of society dictating whether people reproduce sexually or asexually. Furthermore, he objects to initiating cloning experiments in humans, fearing that the first trials could breed a monstrosity (19). One also has to wonder about the psychosocial consequences of producing clonants. A firm and unique sense of identity may be difficult to achieve if one sees a thousand genetic carbon copies of oneself. However, man may derive comfort from knowing that he can achieve complete genetic immortality. In the future social class may become more a function of reproductive status than of economic status. Although it is a long way from a laboratory of cloned frogs to a civilization of cloned people, it is not too early to consider the implications of this research.

All of these developments, from using hormones to cloning men, may radically alter the process and meaning of reproduction; we are entering an era in which a total dissociation of sexuality and procreation is possible. If this occurs, some believe it will inevitably lead to the obsolescence of the family. This prediction is a new twist on an old theme. Lester Frank Ward, Charlotte Perkins Gilman, and Thorstein Veblen, among others, felt that the family would be superseded by technology—its economic functions by the factory, its educational functions by the school,

and its reproductive functions by the laboratory (24). Nevertheless, despite technology's alleged assault upon the integrity of the
family, the family persists. Innovations in reproductive procedures
may alter the roles of its members, such as allowing women a
greater choice of careers. If there will be a gradually increasing
separation between life-giving and love-making, the emotional
and sexual *expectations* between husband and wife may become
redefined. But saying the family will change is quite different
from saying it will disappear. Regardless of how the family of
tomorrow will be constituted, its psychological function—that is,
generating a sense of belonging and identity among its members
—will remain for many years to come. Advancements in reproductive techniques may result, not in the abolition of the
family, but rather in the alteration of its activities and objectives.

Genetic control. Estimates have been made that 25 percent of all
hospital beds are occupied by patients whose physical and emotional disorders are partially genetic in origin (25). The ability to
correct these diseases by directly altering the patient's genetic
endowment has, at least until recently, alluded medical science.
All a physician can do is to inform parents of a genetically diseased
child about the possible risks of a subsequent child having a
similar condition. In the not too distant future, however, this
relative therapeutic impotence may be rectified.

   In the past 20 years many discoveries, such as deciphering the
chemical structure of DNA and synthesizing a biologically active
viral gene, have laid the groundwork for successful genetic
modification. Another significant advance has been the use of
amniocentesis to identify the genetic makeup of a fetus. In this
procedure a hollow needle is inserted through the mother's
abdominal and uterine walls and into the amniotic sac, and fluid
and cells shed by the fetus are withdrawn. These cells can be
stained and photographed to produce a karyotype, or a picture of
the subject's chromosomes arranged in a standardized order. This
technique allows the physician to visualize directly the chromosomes of the fetus and thereby to identify the existence of some

genetic disorders prior to birth. If the karyotype indicates that the child will probably be defective, the parents may choose to abort the fetus.

Amniocentesis and karyotyping may provide a humanitarian alternative to the status quo. Advocates argue that these techniques will save parents from the anguish of raising a defective child, will free society from the burden of supporting it, and will rescue children from the pain of a degrading existence (17). Others ask if parents, doctors, or society has the right to determine who shall or shall not be admitted to the human community. According to Marc Lappé, "It would be unthinkable and immoral if in our zeal to 'conquer' genetic defects, we failed to recognize that the 'defectives' we identify and abort are no less human than we" (26, p. 9).

Although some parents will know in advance that their child will be defective, they may still want to have him. In these cases the possibility of social coercion may arise. As Bruce Hilton points out, "The sympathy toward parents 'afflicted' with a mongoloid child will change in the day when we know they *chose* to have the child" (27, p. 9) (Hilton's italics).

This concern presupposes that one can always and clearly distinguish the genetically healthy from the genetically defective individual. In reality, however, the diagnosis of "genetic health" is a relative one. Almost everyone carries at least one lethal recessive gene. Furthermore, the same gene that partially protects an individual from one disease may render him more susceptible to another disease. In the United States if two individuals mated who had sickle cell trait (a genetically determined abnormal hemoglobin), they could give birth to a child with sickle cell anemia, a painful and always fatal disorder. However, if the same two people with sickle cell trait lived in West Africa, their chances for survival would be enhanced because sickle cell trait provides protection from malaria. Are these individuals genetically healthy? The answer to this question depends as much upon geography as it does upon genetics (28). Some abnormal genes may lead to difficulties *only* under the influence of certain external conditions. For instance, under most circumstances men who carry a defective gene for an enzyme abbreviated G6PD will be completely asymptomatic. However, by ingesting aspirin they may contract a serious, if not fatal, anemia (29). Although a fetus with this condition would be genetically defective, most parents would not choose to abort it. Without taking aspirin, the individual could live a long and healthy life.

Finally, when practitioners become highly sophisticated in interpreting karyotypes, they may be able to determine not only the clearly abnormal fetus, but the *optimal* one as well (26). Therefore, parents, in their quest for the "perfect" offspring, could conceivably choose to abort a normal child. All of this suggests that in the future genetics rather than religion may most vividly confront man with the eternal questions of the meaning and purpose of life.

Some experts believe that man's genetic future is in peril. They argue that medical advances have preserved genes that otherwise would have been eliminated by natural selection and that the expanded use of nuclear energy, radiation emitting devices (e.g., X-rays, microwave ovens), medications, and chemical additives will increase mutation rates. Ramsey predicts that some future generation may experience 20 percent genetic deaths, and those who manage to survive will be seriously burdened by the responsibility of supporting a genetically inferior species (30).

More optimistic experts maintain that tampering with the present gene pool to avert some possible future disaster may be both unnecessary and ill-advised. They argue that even if Ramsey's forecast materializes, it will not occur for many hundreds, if not thousands of years. Although we have no way of knowing in advance, because the world of tomorrow will most likely require different genetic characteristics than the world of today, currently deleterious genes may have a positive survival advantage in the future (31). Consequently, they believe that given our present lack of knowledge, aggressive programs that attempt to improve man's genetic endowment may be unwarranted and in the long run possibly even dangerous. In the interim they propose that less drastic solutions be discovered that will prevent a future genetic catastrophe. For example, to be hairless may have once been a disadvantage, but with the invention of clothes this danger was overcome. Medical as well as other environmental innovations may act in a similar way in the future without placing an undue burden upon society. They also point out that civilization would do better to worry about the immediate specter of a nuclear or ecological holocaust than to become hysterical over some cataclysm that may or may not occur in the distant future (32–33). In contrast, however, others maintain that more active solutions must be devised, and devised now, if our species is to survive. Unfortunately, nobody agrees on the best method to avoid the degeneration of the gene pool. For the most part three different approaches—*euphenics*, *genetic manipulation*, and *eugenics*—have been advocated.

Many believe that *euphenics* is the most immediate and promising of these alternatives (31–32, 34). It can be defined as the modification or control of the expression of existing genes in order to lead to a desirable phenotype (34).* A great deal of contemporary medical practice is a form of euphenic modification. For example, by administering insulin to diabetics the physician seeks to correct the genetic defect partially responsible for the disorder. Another current application of euphenics involves restricting the dietary intake of substances that cause genotypically abnormal individuals to produce harmful bodily chemicals. For example, phenylketonuria is a rare inherited disorder that leads to severe mental retardation. Patients with this condition are unable to metabolize the amino acid phenylalamine; therefore, most doctors prescribe a phenylalamine-free diet. Although euphenic interventions are relatively safe, they fail to reverse what many believe to be mankind's perpetually declining genetic

---

* A genotype can be defined as the fundamental hereditary constitution of the organism. A phenotype is the observable hereditary characteristics of the organism that arise from an interaction of the genotype with the environment. For example, if a patient with a genetic G6PD deficiency abstains from aspirin and a few other potentially dangerous substances, he would be genotypically abnormal but phenotypically normal. However, if the same individual would ingest aspirin, and thereby develop an anemia, he would be both genotypically and phenotypically symptomatic.

endowment. As long as medically treated genotypically aberrant individuals continue to procreate, their defective genes will be transmitted to future generations.

However, various forms of *genetic manipulation* may avert this dilemma. These techniques include extracting deleterious genes, supplying missing genes, and altering simultaneously a whole block of characteristics. Although these procedures may be accomplished in many conceivable ways, one possibility would be to use fine beams of radiation to slice through the DNA molecule or to delete segments of it. Alternatively, "repressor molecules" may be developed that would embed themselves upon selected portions of the DNA chain to inhibit the expression of their harmful effects. Viruses could supply genetic material missing from the chromosome. If these and other techniques can be utilized before fertilization or at the very earliest stages of embryonic development, scientists may be able to fashion individuals devoid of genetic defects or endowed with certain predetermined specifications (2, 32, 35).

Until now these techniques have been applied to simple and primitive forms of life, such as bacteria. They certainly will not be applied to man in the immediate future, if ever. Nevertheless, because human genetic manipulation is theoretically possible, eventually it may be utilized. Although the initial reason for its use may be therapeutic, ultimately these procedures may enable man to design his species. He may create superior scholars, athletes, or warriors. Whether we possess the wisdom to make appropriate decisions, however, remains to be seen.

In *The Republic* Plato suggests, "The best of either sex should be united with the best as often, and the inferior with the inferior, as seldom as possible" (36, p. 158). Two millennia later this guideline is still embodied in eugenic thought. *Eugenics* can be defined as the selection and recombination of genes already existing in the gene pool of a population (34). Sometimes eugenics is divided roughly into its "positive" and "negative" forms. The former entails the mating of genetically normal or superior individuals. Herman Muller, one of its leading exponents, believes that we could reduce "the problem of creeping genetic deterioration" by using AID with healthy stored spermatozoa (37). Before an effective, positive eugenics program could be launched, however, the presence of deleterious genes in a phenotypically normal person would have to be identified (34). Even if this can be accomplished, two questions remain: Which genetic traits ought to be sustained, and who should make that decision? Muller believes that cooperativeness and general intelligence are the two qualities most worthy of preservation (37). Nevertheless, these factors may be as much a product of environment as they are of heredity. Moreover, others may nominate different characteristics. There also is the danger that in selecting criteria the choosers may be unduly swayed by currently popular opinions and act hastily in ways that ultimately would be detrimental to the species. Because the social and biological requirements of societies perpetually evolve, a gene that is valuable in one century may be lethal in another century (31–32).

Negative eugenics attempt to eliminate deleterious genes by preventing those with undesirable traits from propagating or by aborting their afflicted offspring. Although patients with hemophilia, sickle cell anemia, phenylketonuria, and Huntington's chorea would definitely be included in this category, others, such as those with juvenile-onset diabetes and schizophrenia, also may be prime candidates for a negative eugenics program. Because tests for some of these conditions already exist, physicians are able to discuss with patients the probable consequences of reproducing. This counselling can help a couple reach a more informed decision about having children. However, because most deleterious genes are transmitted by genotypically defective but phenotypically normal (i.e., heterozygous) individuals, many believe that ultimately negative eugenics programs will be unable to reverse man's declining genetic pool (31–32). Furthermore, would one want to dissuade a Brahms, who happens to have schizophrenia, from mating? Because predicting how genes will combine and recombine is difficult, by extinguishing a defective gene a superior gene also may be eliminated. An apocryphal vignette tells of how Isadora Duncan proposed to George Bernard

Shaw by proclaiming, "Think of a child with my body and your mind." Shaw declined the offer and explained, "Ah, but suppose it had *my* body and *your* mind" (2)!

Until we have a much fuller understanding of heredity, eugenic programs will be unable to forestall mankind's deteriorating genetic pool. Even if this knowledge is available, as undoubtedly it will be someday, social resistance may inhibit people from practicing what Ramsey calls an "ethic of genetic duty" (30). If eugenics are utilized, most authorities believe that participation must be voluntary (30, 32); to do otherwise would be unethical. However, because in our society procreation is viewed as an inalienable right (38), leaving the option of practicing an ethic of genetic duty up to the individual may result in many choosing to reproduce despite the potential consequences. Thus, a voluntary program may have a minimal effect upon the overall gene pool.

Paul Ramsey suggests that underlying the many pathways genetic research could follow are four interrelated and fundamental ethical questions. Can man ever be expected to possess the intellect and wisdom necessary to direct his own evolutionary future? Will medicine's inventive use of genetic technology destroy parenthood as a basic task of humanity? Does man's deliberate attempt to modify radically his genetic constitution represent a dangerous aspiration toward Godhood? Will geneticists' efforts to improve humanity paradoxically and inevitably lead to species suicide (19)? These questions will necessitate continued and extensive examination, if wisdom will guide our evolutionary destiny.

Regulation of Behavior. Because all perceptions, thoughts, feelings, and activities are mediated through the brain, the neuropathologist Santiago Ramón y Cajal observed, "As long as our brain is a mystery, the universe, the reflection of the structure of the brain, will also be a mystery" (36, p. 45). Thus, neurophysiologic research will not only enhance our understanding of the brain, but also of the world that interacts with it. The belief in the mind-body dualism of old has been superseded by the recognition that all cognition, perception, and behavior is the product of a complex interaction between genetic, physiologic, and environmental influences. Therefore, to treat psychobiological diseases, physicians focus upon both "talking" and biological treatments. In comparison to verbal therapies (e.g., psychoanalysis, group therapy), biological interventions (e.g., medication, electroconvulsive therapy, electrical stimulation of the brain, psychosurgery) have generated a tempest of public and professional alarm (39–40). Efforts to expand our understanding of the brain are often viewed as diabolical schemes being perpetrated by cold-blooded scientists upon innocent victims. Probably no other area of biomedical research has aroused so much misunderstanding, irrationality, and consternation. It must be placed within a reasonable perspective.

Before the birth of Christ, Lucretius wrote that "the mind like a sick body can be healed and changed by medicine" (36, p. 311). Not until the 20th century has this belief become a clinical reality. Drugs have been developed that are usually effective in the treatment of schizophrenia, depression, mania, anxiety, and epilepsy. Compounds such as LSD and mescaline can enduce a transitory psychosis. The discovery of these psychoactive agents has kindled the expectation that other chemicals can be synthesized that could modify every aspect of human behavior. Pessimists warn that eventually drugs will rob men of their individuality and "free will." They fear that under the guise of benevolence, doctors will use their newfound chemical power to exact conformity from their patients and to mask symptoms caused by social ills rather than by personal difficulties. According to this argument, medications will be administered to suppress dissent and to divert attention from social inequities and injustices (41). What frightens some critics the most is that people on drugs will be unable to realize they are being controlled and, therefore, will not only fail to resist taking these medications, but may actually enjoy doing so (42).

These estimations contain elements of the truth and of the absurd. Psychoactive agents that can regulate many types of human behavior and experience will be discovered. Medications could be used to stifle legitimate deviance and to divert attention from the social causes of mental illness. However, the same criticisms could be leveled against "talking" therapies, which could, in a way, be considered more insidious. Because an elaborate social, educational, and legal structure has been erected, only physicians have the skill and authority to administer medications, but *anyone* can legally practice psychotherapy. Furthermore, whereas many psychotherapy patients are unaware of the subtle coercion taking place, medicated individuals usually know they are being affected by drugs (43). If people do not wish to take medications, under most circumstances they can refuse to do so. Various studies of hospitalized psychiatric patients reveal that 5 to 63 percent of them fail to take their prescribed drugs (44).

Some experts have argued that the effects of psychotherapy are more benign than those of medications, because the effectiveness of the latter is greater than that of the former (40). If true, this is hardly reassuring; it suggests that psychotherapy patients are paying for a treatment of lesser value, which in and of itself raises many serious ethical questions (45). More importantly, because *all* of us induce people to behave in ways that are favorable to ourselves, everyone practices a kind of social coercion. Because these pressures are exerted by teachers, bosses, advertisers, relatives, and friends, they are a *normal part of everyday life*. We are often unable to identify these pressures, or worse yet, believe they are nonexistent (46). Although coercion by medication exists, it is more overt and, therefore, possibly less dangerous than social coercion which creates the illusion that it is nonexistent.

I am not suggesting that the presence of social coercion justifies the use of chemical coercion. Instead, I am proposing that *all* forms of behavioral control must be identified specifically and regulated appropriately. Because of the seeming "invisibility" of social coercion, it, rather than medications, will always exert the greatest influence upon man's behavior. The responses of a medicated patient are the product of not only the drug itself, but also of the individual's personality and environment. Truth serum cannot make a person tell the truth; antipsychotic medications cannot rob a patient of his psychosis. There is a tendency to ascribe power to drugs, which in reality they fail to possess. Although many believe that medications exert the same effect on everyone, no such uniformity exists. Because of neurological and psychological differences among people, there is a great variability of responses among those who take psychotropic agents. From a pharmacological perspective, the fear that some future demagogue could pollute the water supply with medications to exact conformity is more in the realm of fiction than fact.

Psychosurgery has been the object of extensive and continued medical and ethical controversy. When first popularized in the 1940s, psychosurgery was expected to calm severely agitated and uncontrollably violent patients by removing or destroying isolated segments of their brains. The initial results were disappointing. Some patients became more excitable; many others became extremely lethargic and intellectually impaired. However, by the 1960s, as neurosurgeons refined their operative techniques and acquired a deeper understanding of neuroanatomy and neurophysiology, interest in psychosurgery became revitalized. Psychosurgery was anticipated to be effective in patients whose destructive behavior was caused by an *identifiable* lesion of the brain, which could *not* be corrected by more conventional therapeutic interventions (47–49), and to reduce excessive tension, anxiety, fear, depression, or obsessions where all other methods had failed (50–52).

Although we cannot yet determine if this renewed enthusiasm is justified, we should examine some of the medical, social, and ethical problems associated with psychosurgery. A frequently voiced concern is that someday the operation will be used extensively against political militants. The chance of this occurring, however, is unlikely. Because psychosurgery is an extremely complex, delicate, and expensive procedure, tyrants would find it to be a highly inefficient way of suppressing dissent. Auschwitz and Buchenwald should remind us that more economical, proficient, and malevolent techniques exist for disposing of political deviants. Another fear is that by means of psychosurgery a future Hitler could transform meek citizens into assaultive soldiers. However, a person whose brain has been surgically altered to cause violent behavior would be unable to restrict his outbursts to politically strategic situations. As Goebbels demonstrated, mass political violence can be elicited by environmental manipulations without having to resort to psychosurgery (47).

Another objection to the surgical modification of behavior is that it deprives the patient of free will, self-control, and human dignity (53). If psychosurgery is applied indiscriminately, this concern is justified. The force of this criticism is weakened, however, upon considering the plight of those who suffer from seizure-induced violence. Usually these individuals are frightened, repulsed, and remorseful about their assaultive behavior; they plead for surgical relief from their symptoms. As a result, neurosurgeon Vernon Mark believes that psychosurgery can give ". . .the patient more, rather than less, control over his own behavior. It enhances, and does not diminish, his dignity. It adds to, and does not detract from, his human qualities" (47, p. 5). Of course the danger always exists that physicians will inappropriately utilize psychosurgery. Although this risk must not be underestimated, we must recognize that conducting any major medical procedure can result in serious consequences. The answer to the problem of the potential misuse of psychosurgery lies not in outlawing its application nor in restricting research in the field, but in carefully monitoring its performance.

One of the major disadvantages of psychosurgery is that once the operation is conducted, its effects are permanent. This irreversibility occurs because destroyed nerve cells are unable to regenerate. However, electrical stimulation of the brain (ESB) may provide an alternative to the treatment of some neurologically produced behavior disorders. The technique often involves implanting filamentous platinum electrodes insulated with teflon into specific deep structures of the brain. These electrodes can remain in place for many years without the patient experiencing any physical discomfort, neurological impairment, or cosmetic embarrassment. The proximal end of the electrode is connected to a two-way radio communication system called a "stimoreceiver" that can transmit electrical impulses both to and from the brain. By stimulating specific parts of the brain ESB already has helped thousands of patients with focal epilepsy, involuntary muscular movements, intractable pain, severe obsessive-compulsive behavior, anxiety neurosis, violence, and other disorders.

Whereas the electroencephalogram can only detect electrical currents emanating from the surface of the brain, ESB allows the physician to gather data from its deeper structures. It often can provide invaluable diagnostic information that is unavailable by more conventional procedures. By linking a stimoreceiver to a computer, a localized electrical discharge announcing the imminence of an epileptic attack is picked up by the implanted electrode and telemetered to and analyzed by a computer. In turn the machine transmits impulses to the brain and aborts the seizure (54–55). In the future ESB may be used for the treatment of anorexia nervosa and persistent insomnia as well as for the understanding of the neurophysiological correlates of mental illnesses (54). Despite the promise offered by ESB, many have expressed alarm over its application.

Perry London argues that ESB represents a dangerous addition to medicine's armamentarium of behavioral control technology. He writes:

> Docility, fearful withdrawal, and panicked efforts at escape can be made to alternate with fury and ferocity of such degree that its subject can as readily destroy himself by exhaustion from his consuming rage as he can the object of it, whom he attacks, heedless of both danger and opportunity. Eating, drinking, sleeping, moving of bowels or limbs or organs of sensation, gracefully or in spastic comedy, can all be managed on electrical demand by puppeteers whose flawless strings are pulled from miles away by the unseen call of radio and whose puppets, made of flesh and blood, look "like electronic toys," so little self-direction do they seem to have (39, p. 137).

Because no amount of intentionality can override an electrical stimulus applied to the brain, London is correct when he says that scientists presently have the ability to elicit these grotesque behaviors. However, the weakness of his argument is that he fails to distinguish between the possibility and the probability of the improper use of ESB. If a despot wishes to torture his opponents, there certainly are easier ways to do so. Although it is conceivable that some convoluted scientists could conceivably get a perverse thrill from watching the bizarre activities of electrically stimulated patients, the probability of this occurring is minimal. Nevertheless, serious risks do exist. To expand his knowledge of cerebral activity, an overzealous investigator may perform ESB in humans without a reasonable possibility that the patient could accrue any substantial benefits from the procedure. Because many people who desperately request ESB already have exhausted hope of obtaining relief from more traditional methods, the scientist, in a moment of excessive compassion, may grant their wish even though the chances of success are highly unlikely. Conversely, because of excessive fears of ESB, some doctors may refuse to use it even though it probably would help the patient. It would be unconscionable to deny ESB to an individual on so called "humanistic" grounds, when the alternative is permanent incarceration in a mental institution or a prison. The answers to these problems do not lie in restricting further research or in mesmerizing the public with lurid portraits of ESB. Instead, the activities of scientists not only require but demand thorough and constant monitoring by those who are knowledgeable of its medical and ethical consequences.

On the more distant horizon, chemical techniques to enhance memory and learning may become available. Although we are a long way from completely understanding the physiological basis of these activities, many believe that ribonucleic acid (RNA) does play a critical role. In the early 1950s planaria were conditioned to contract after receiving a stimulus from a bright light. When they were pulverized and fed to a breed of untrained cannibalistic planaria, the untrained flatworms acquired the conditioned properties of the trained planaria. Other experiments have suggested that RNA is the critical substance responsible for the transfer of memory in these animals. Although what applies to worms does not necessarily apply to humans, the opportunity of understanding the processes by which memory can be stored and transferred raises intriguing possibilities. In the remote future eating could replace teaching as a major educational vehicle. As Gordon Taylor notes, "Professors of psychology, half seriously, envisaged the day when their class would learn their subjects by eating their teachers" (2, p. 139). Another possibility would be if, by ingesting RNA from animals, man would be able to learn from and about animal experiences. Techniques may be developed that would prevent learning and erase memory. Studies have shown that if the antibiotic puromycin is administered to goldfish shortly after they have learned a task, the goldfish are unable to remember what they have been taught. It also has been found that 8-azaguanine can prevent the synthesis of RNA, and thereby, could theoretically inhibit memory formation (2). Both of these findings suggest that drugs capable of obliterating a person's memory could be created. The potential misuse of these chemicals by political groups raises momentous ethical problems.

Although an enriching and stimulating environment is necessary for intellectual growth, eventually biological techniques may also be capable of raising intelligence. Experts contend that within the forseeable future transforming a moron into a genius would be unlikely, and they generally agree that once an individual's neurological tissues mature, increasing his intelligence would be difficult. Nevertheless, within the next 50 years it might be possible that procedures utilized during prenatal development could enhance a person's intellectual potential (17, 56–57). Although how this will occur is difficult to forecast, several alternative methods may be applied. As the relationship between heredity and I.Q. is clarified, genetic manipulations could potentially enhance intelligence. Experiments have shown that when pregnant rats and frogs are injected with growth hormone, they produce offspring with larger brains and greater learning abilities. There also are tentative indications that by simultaneously reducing atmospheric pressure upon a pregnant mother's abdomen and increasing the oxygen flow to the fetus, the baby's intellectual capacity can be augmented. One child born under these conditions was able to answer the telephone at 13 months and to speak four languages by the age of three. This child might have been exceptional even if exposed to normal prenatal influences. However, other children raised by this method have demonstrated similar intellectual skills (2). If these and other biological interventions will be capable of raising intellectual levels, the implications for the future of man are enormous.

In large measure, the social consequences of physiologically enhancing intelligence may depend upon who would benefit the most from these procedures. A powerful intellectual elite could be developed, if only the IQs of brighter individuals were elevated. Although this possibility may be frightening to many, all societies, whether medieval, capitalist, or communist, have a ruling elite. Therefore, the question is not whether such an elite exists, but rather if it should be based upon ecclesiastical power, physical brutality, economic strength, political cunning, or intellectual ability. One could argue that the latter quality would be preferable. Yet many fear that such an elite would oppress those with lesser intellectual capabilities. This supposition is based on the widely held assumption that there is an inverse relation between intellect and compassion. However, studies indicate that no such correlation, either positive or negative, exists (58). My own bias is that since the existence of an elite is historically inevitable, I would prefer it to be comprised of intelligent people. However, since I see myself as being intelligent, this view is admittedly suspect; we tend to value those characteristics which we ourselves possess (59).

Another possibility is that only those with lower IQs would benefit from techniques aimed at raising intelligence. Undoubtedly, this greater intellectual equality would profoundly affect man's psychology and social institutions. A further alternative would be that different types of intellectual skills would be affected by these biological interventions. Verbal competence might be elevated in some and performance abilities in others. Once again, the important questions are who will get what raised and who will make the determination (57)?

Aging.   Most of the anticipated biomedical innovations discussed in this chapter may contribute to the prolongation of life. Although this objective has been valued since antiquity, the mere postponement of death is a mixed blessing. When Gulliver traveled and met the Struttlebugs, he soon discovered that eternal life and eternal youth are very different. There is little value in prolonging one's existence, if that existence is to be filled with infirmities, misery, and despair.

As discussed earlier, most authorities believe that aging results from a random and progressive death of individual cells that eventually affects the entire body. To reverse this process several approaches have been considered. Organ transplantation already has been mentioned. Another technique involves the use of cortisone and testosterone. Some elderly men who were injected with these hormones were able to increase their muscular strength by as much as 47 percent. Unfortunately, these drugs have numerous side-effects, and therefore, many problems will have to be overcome before they could play a useful role in rejuvenating tissues (2). Prehoda has speculated that cloned cells could be substituted for devitalized ones. Because dying cells are replaced by fibrous connective tissue, this procedure would necessitate breaking up connective tissue (60). Despite the possible applications of all of these techniques, a major physiologic reversal of the aging process may not be discovered for many years.

Although the average American life span has increased from 47.3 years in 1900 to 71.2 years in 1972 (61), there are indications that this trend is beginning to plateau (60). If so, new discoveries will be necessary to extend man's longevity. Until these advances are developed, most of us will passively accept the seeming inevitability of death; most of us, that is, except for people like Robert Ettinger. He claims that by freezing recently deceased individuals, at present they can be preserved indefinitely with minimal tissue deterioration. If we accept Ettinger's hypothesis,

. . . we need only arrange to have our bodies, *after we die*, stored in suitable freezers against the time when science may be able to help us. No matter what kills us, whether old age or disease, and even if freezing techniques are still crude when we die, *sooner or later* our friends of the future should be equal to the task of reviving and curing us (62, p. 15). (Ettinger's italics).

As of 1973, 14 individuals have been frozen (60) at the approximate cost of $42,200 each (2). Currently, medical opinion is divided as to whether this procedure will only produce human Popsicles or provide mankind with his first genuine opportunity for immortality. If Ettinger is correct, however, cryogenic preservation will have some intriguing—if not chilling—ramifications.

Individuals would have a chance to live in the world of their great-great-great-grandchildren. Depending upon if they like what they see, they could immediately return to the ice box or continue to live above ground. At the same time, their relatives may have a variety of feelings about resurrecting their frozen ancestors. Considering how some people enjoy tracing their family trees, think how exciting it could be for them if that tree came to life. Alternatively, others may be less enthusiastic, fearing that they may have to relinquish part of their inheritance or get stuck supporting the new (or old?) arrival. If cryo-burials replaced traditional ones, eventually the ratio of frozen to living bodies would become enormous. In time it may be difficult to find enough people capable of maintaining the "refrigitoriums." Furthermore, could a frozen person be revived against his will if he was needed to testify in court or to clarify an historical dispute? The issues that could be raised are inexhaustible, and cryogenic preservation derives its special fascination partially from this fact.

Prehoda eschews the "freeze now" approach, believing that hibernation would be a more feasible scientific objective (63). Whereas cryogenic preservation entails a complete cessation of bodily processes, hibernation involves a slowing of physiological activities. Experiments with hamsters have shown that hibernation is partially under genetic control. By utilizing the genetic manipulation techniques described earlier, man could be endowed with the ability to hibernate. However, one need not resort to these complicated and potentially dangerous techniques. Because genes produce enzymes, which in turn control the synthesis of proteins, these enzymes and proteins could be isolated and injected into humans to induce hibernation. The potential applications of hibernation are numerous. It could alleviate the boredom of long distance space travel. In case of a nuclear war, lead-shielded hibernacula could be used to offer the survivors protection from radiation. If hibernation replaced sleep, the slowing of physiological processes that result from the former could theoretically prolong the viability of bodily organs and, therefore, life itself (2). Whether any of these possibilities will materialize remains to be seen. Nevertheless, Prehoda believes that "generous research funding could be the catalyst permitting early success, thereby allowing many readers to travel into the exotic world of Century 21 as hibernauts and cryonauts" (63, p. xv).

COPING WITH THE NEW BIOLOGY.   As scientific advances unfold, many exclaim that we are entering upon the threshold of a biological armageddon. Premonitions abound—innovations in reproduction will subvert the family, transplantation of organs will destroy man's identity, genetic manipulation will extinguish the species, and behavioral control will undermine human dignity. We are told that in the future ". . . manual workers will have exoskeletons, athletes will have spare hearts, and computer programmers spare heads" (2, p. 93). Only by taking a pill ". . . will people be happy or sad, amiable or aggressive, active or lazy, calm or anxious. . ." (2, p. 133). Rosenfeld suggests that someday women may enter a supermarket and, as if purchasing a package of seeds, will select a day-old frozen embryo enclosed in a colorful wrapper illustrating what its adult form will resemble (2). *Esquire* depicts legless astronauts specially bred for long-term space voyages, cloned Mahalia Jacksons and Joe Namaths for entertainment, and men with prehensile feet and tails hanging onto planets with low gravitational pulls (19). As the prophets of doom project their ominous and grotesque visions, the oracles of humanism cry that unless the biomedical revolution is stopped, a catastrophe of cataclysmic proportions will be inevitable. Of course, not everybody writes about the new biology with lurid sensationalism. Many intelligent and thoughtful men have expressed concern over the potential consequences of biomedical innovations. Alarmed by these developments and by their accompanying social and ethical dilemmas, they seek a moratorium on biomedical experimentation and implementation.

In contrast to these perspectives I would suggest the following: (a) The widespread fear of biomedical innovations derives largely from developments other than the specific projected biological discoveries themselves. (b) The continual forecasting of dire predictions will inhibit man from coping effectively with the consequences of biomedical research. (c) There is a tendency to exaggerate the dangers of the biomedical revolution. I believe that whatever difficulties will emerge can be resolved. (d) To attempt to halt completely biomedical investigations or to prevent totally the clinical application of these findings is fruitless. (e) Individuals, not society, must assume the responsibility for their actions vis-à-vis the new biology by adopting a sense of personal ethical accountability.

I would maintain that the widespread concern, if not trepidation, over the anticipated biomedical revolution is rooted in man's perceptions and distortions of time, change, and science. Undoubtedly, almost everyone who reads about a panorama of exotic biomedical innovations would become alarmed initially. It would be akin to the bewildering experience of suddenly awakening to find oneself in the year 2175. The fright sensed by this individual would not result primarily from the nature of his newly discovered world *per se*, but rather from having been deprived of 200 years to acclimate himself to it. Similarly, the dismay generated by discussions of the new biology derives largely from the illusion that all of these innovations will occur at almost the same time, * thereby overwhelming the reader with an avalanche of dilemmas

---

* The expected dates of occurrence for many potential biomedical developments are enumerated in Appendix B.

for which he, at least psychologically, has been inadequately prepared. In reality, however, because the discoveries previously alluded to will be introduced over a period of centuries, rather than all at once, time will soften their impact. Therefore, the irrational fear created by portraits of man's biological future can be reduced by remembering that humanity will have the opportunity to acclimate and adjust themselves to these changes as they gradually evolve.

Although what Taylor calls "The Biological Time Bomb" (2) will not explode all at once, its very existence implies that the status quo will lose its stability. Man is frightened by change, especially when he cannot exactly predict its ultimate form. Because he does not know precisely where the biomedical revolution will eventually lead, his concern tends to escalate into alarm. Man's concern over the new biology derives in large measure from a fear of change and especially the *prospect* of change.

Because people in our society tend to distrust science and scientists, the anxiety generated by the uncertainty of our biological futures becomes aggravated even further. Believing that his fate was determined primarily by the will of the Lord, pre-17th-century man reserved his most passionate blessings and blasphemies for God. Subsequently, in one of those Copernican turns of history, man began to entrust his destiny to social institutions. In the process he also transferred his hopes and hostilities to them (64). As central figures in this cultural transformation, scientists offended the classical theological establishment (65), and people became divided in their feelings toward science. To some it promised to deliver man from the stagnation of the Middle Ages; to others it threatened the status quo. Today science has replaced God as the recipient of man's highest expectations and deepest resentments. Our secular society assumes that science will perform miracles, and when it fails to do so or when its schemes go awry, men quickly become disillusioned and suspicious of it. Since Hiroshima this trend has become accentuated so that science is viewed by many with skepticism, if not with outright hostility. That biological experimentation becomes the object of popular antagonism and alarm is not surprising. Like their Renaissance counterparts, contemporary biologists are accused of "aspiring to Godhood" (19) by undermining our traditional norms, values, and ethics. Thus, the hysteria and consternation frequently characterizing discussions of the new biology reflect more than simply a concern over the specific innovations themselves. Instead, their fears often represent a more global animosity toward and distrust of science and especially scientists.

By expressing excessive alarm over the potential consequences of the new biology, critics believe they are rendering a valuable public service. Their efforts, however, may have exactly the opposite effect. There are many dangers in making dire predictions. (a) People are becoming so inundated with the proliferation of doomsday forecasts that a "boy who cried wolf" mentality is emerging. Society is becoming so desensitized to ominous projections that when a *real* crisis does arise, nobody may recognize or care about it (66). (b) The public may respond to dire pronouncements by hastily and unthoughtfully instituting inexpedient programs. What initially appears as a short-term gain may turn out to be a long-range disaster (67). (c) When confronted with an anticipated crisis, many expend their energies discovering a scapegoat instead of seeking a rational solution. (d) Even if the problem is a genuine one and people respond constructively to it, they may become so preoccupied with the crisis that they could overlook other dilemmas urgently in need of attention. (e) By excessively focusing upon the alleged potential dangers of biomedical experimentation society may not fully consider the dangers of *not* proceeding with such research. (f) The public may believe the problem is of such overwhelming magnitude and complexity that it would be impossible ever to find an answer. Faced with what they are convinced is an insurmountable dilemma society may choose to avoid it altogether. If this occurs, not only are the problems ignored, but people's faith in their ability to manage a complex society becomes shaken even further. After being perpetually confronted with their inability to contend with supposedly cataclysmic developments, man could adopt a "what's the use" attitude. Why bother healing the sick, teaching the young, or helping the poor if doomsday is just around the corner? Instead of leading to an active search for constructive solutions, the continual rendering of dire predictions could immobilize society in a nihilistic quagmire (68).

Proclamations of impending catastrophes inhibit the public's ability to respond effectively to genuine problems, and the critics themselves appear stalemated by their own dire forecasts. Their proposals often reflect their own pessimism and despair. Generally speaking, their basic message can be summarized as follows: "The dangers posed by the biomedical revolution are so monumentous that until their ethical and social problems have been fully resolved, we must severely restrict, if not absolutely prohibit, all further research into these areas." Even if one accepts the dubious premise that the new biology will devastate society, their recommendation leaves much to be desired. The efficacy of this nonsolution is like attempting to stop a stampeding herd of buffalo with a traffic light.

A moratorium on biomedical investigations is impossible to implement. Although many authors, including scientists themselves, insist that controversial biological research must stop (2, 19, 21, 24, 39, 69–70), nobody stops. Because few scientists believe that their own research is ethically irresponsible, they are unlikely to discontinue their own research, especially when it could lead to a significant breakthrough—not to mention personal fame and fortune. In an ethically pluralistic society what may be considered reprehensible by some may be viewed favorably by others. Furthermore, cultural values change quickly and radically. Within the past decade the public has become increasingly tolerant of abortion and even AID (17, 71). Yet, whereas the United States Congress recently passed legislation promoting family planning (71), they also banned experimentation on any "living" human fetus (72). The clash between the "old morality" and the "new morality" is producing a society in which ethical norms are in continual flux. Even if one standard exists, it still is difficult to distinguish between what is or is not ethically acceptable. Although many universities and hospitals establish committees that are supposed to ensure that experiments carried out within their own institutions meet certain ethical criteria, these committees hardly can be expected to halt completely controversial research. Their authority usually covers only investigations performed on human subjects. Animal experimentation is rarely inhibited, and most ethically dubious innovations are first discovered with animals.

Because the end results of research cannot be predicted, experiments initially untainted by ethical doubts may lead accidentally to highly controversial findings. For instance, knowledge of cloning may be enhanced as a by-product of research primarily intended to devise improved methods of contraception (71). Consequently, regulation by funding agencies or ethics committees cannot prevent secondary discoveries from being made. Even if the United States government *could* terminate *all* controversial biological research—a highly unlikely prospect—what would prevent British, Russian, or Chinese investigators from pursuing this work? Clearly, the issue is global rather than national in scope.

Recognizing the impossibility of preventing research, some critics have suggested that better control could be exerted by restricting the *implementation* of controversial discoveries (73–74). In reality, however, when the time comes to apply these findings in humans, there often are justifiable reasons for doing so. For example, artificial insemination was initially a highly controversial procedure. Nevertheless, when it was the only way a couple could have children, there were many ethically sound arguments for utilizing the technique (17). Although legal prohibitions could restrict the execution of controversial procedures in humans, they are of limited value in two major respects—speed and scope. The law responds rather than anticipates scientific discoveries; when it does respond, it responds slowly (75). By the time legislation is passed, the controversial technique may already have been accepted by, if not applied to, large segments of the population. Even if Congress prohibited the use of certain procedures, they could be performed in other nations (67, 71). Antiabortion laws illustrate the futility of attempting to prevent the implementation of controversial medical interventions. The wealthy simply went to other countries for abortions. The poor obtained illegal and often dangerous abortions within the United States. Although society can reduce, they can never completely inhibit research or prevent the implementation of its discoveries.

I am *not* suggesting that all laboratory and clinical investigations can be justified ethically, nor do I wish to imply that science, left to its own devices, will always benefit mankind. (I expect that very serious mistakes will continue to be made.) What I am proposing is that the general and scientific communities must come to the painful recognition that the biomedical revolution is inevitable. However well intentioned, clarion calls for social responsibility will not prevent scientific innovation. Instead of wasting time issuing ringing "stop research" declarations, we need to focus our energies, both personal and collective, upon coping effectively with inevitable biological discoveries. Each layman, scientist, and clinician must decide if his own ethical standards are consistent with taking advantage of and performing new biomedical techniques. I believe that for a person to decide *on his own* not to participate in unethical procedures is more virtuous than to be prevented from doing so by the Church or the state. At the same time the political, educational, religious, medical, and scientific communities, must explain the nature of these controversial biomedical advances and provide forums for adequate discussion of their ethical and social implications. The full responsibility for this task cannot be placed on physicians and biologists. Although they could and should contribute their technical expertise, evidence indicates that they are no more sophisticated or knowledgeable about social and ethical issues than are laymen (65, 76).

Discussions ought to occur in many arenas of social discourse. Rather than hearing lectures on the mating habits of the centipede, high school science classes should focus upon man's biological future. Television, newspapers, and journals such as *The Hastings Center Report* also could help to inform the public. Thus, society's chief role vis-à-vis the new biology ought to be an educational one.

It would be mistaken, however, to place undue reliance upon society to help us survive the biomedical revolution. We tend to blame society for all kinds of human afflictions from alienation to racism. This approach is an emotionally convenient method of scapegoating, because by saying we are all guilty, none of us are guilty. Worse yet, by accusing everyone, nobody is really held accountable for their actions. By abdicating personal responsibility we expect some ill-defined entity called "society" to rectify the problem. But what is society? It is a collection of individuals and institutions, none of whom has the ability to halt effectively biomedical progress. Legal interventions are slow and limited, scientific restrictions are incomplete, and theological arguments lack authority. The decision to utilize biomedical techniques will inevitably rest with individuals and not with society. The only viable approach is that a norm of *personal* ethical accountability be fostered. For example, instead of asking if society should permit, let us say, *in vitro* fertilization, to ask, "Would *I* have a child by means of *in vitro* fertilization?" would be more constructive and honest. In the very near future it may be possible to determine the sex of a fetus with 90 percent accuracy (56, 77). This could lead to a situation where some individuals would choose to abort a fetus having a sex other than the one they prefer. Instead of asking if society or medicine should allow this to occur, I believe it would be preferable to ask, "Would *I* abort a fetus of undesired sex? If so, under what circumstances?" Society can inform, but men must decide.

By rejecting the utility of issuing dire predictions, refusing to call for a halt of biomedical research and the clinical application of these discoveries, and releasing society from the responsibility of controlling the biomedical revolution, I may be accused of exhibiting the same kind of self-righteousness and arrogance that allegedly has been displayed by the scientific and medical communities for so many years. However, in formulating approaches to cope with the social and ethical consequences of the new biology, I believe suggesting workable notions is better than extolling noble-sounding nonsolutions. By advocating that we need to promote a norm of personal ethical accountability, I hope to focus responsibility where it must belong. We cannot rely upon others to solve the problem. We must assume personal responsibility for coping with the biomedical revolution by preparing ourselves and our children for man's biological destiny.

My opposition to social, legal, and theologically imposed restrictions of the development and use of biomedical innovations does not rest solely upon pragmatic considerations. If we are forced to follow absolute ethical standards that are not adjusted to historical change or individual need, our capacity to cope effectively with the future will be undermined. Any human or social system that cannot incorporate change inevitably atrophies (78). One does not enhance individual dignity by usurping the dignity of individual choice, nor can ethical decisions be made without considering the circumstances surrounding them (17). Although the use of AID may be justified for a man with a low sperm count, it may be unwarranted for a man with a normal sperm count. Similarly, an abortion may be "right" for a woman with eight starving children, but "wrong" for a woman without children. We cannot and will not increase man's sense of free will by depriving him of the freedom to make his own ethical decisions.

NOTES

1. Jonsen, A. R. (1973). "The Totally Implantable Artificial Heart." *Hastings Center Report*, 3(5):1–4.

2. Taylor, G. R. (1969). *The Biological Time Bomb*. New York: New American Library.

3. Latham, A. (1975). "Replaceable You." *New York*, 8(6):37–44.

4. Humphrey, J. H. (1972). "Some Implications of Modern Immunology." In W. Fuller (ed.), *The Biological Revolution: Social Good or Social Evil?* Garden City, N. J.: Doubleday. Pp. 147–165.

5. Longmore, D. (1968). "Implants or Transplants?" *Science Journal*, 4(2): 78–83.

6. Starzl, T. E. (1967). "Ethical Problems in Organ Transplantation: A Clinician's Point of View." *Annals of Internal Medicine*, 67(3) Part II, Supplement 7:32–36.

7. Robertson, R. D., and S. W. Jacob (1968). "The Significance and Future of Organ Banking." *Lex et Scientia*, 5:25–35.

8. *Footnotes to the Future* (1974). "Harvesting the Dead," 4(8):3.

9. Ramsey, P. (1969). "On Updating Death." In D. R. Cutler (ed.), *Updating Life and Death: Essays in Ethics and Medicine.* Boston: Beacon. Pp. 31–54.

10. Beecher, H. K. (1969). "A Definition of Irreversible Coma." In D. R. Cutler (ed.), *Updating Life and Death: Essays in Ethics and Medicine.* Boston: Beacon. Pp. 55–63.

11. National Academy of Sciences, Board on Medicine (1968). "Cardiac Transplantation in Man." *NAS-NRC-NAE News Report,* 18)March):1–3.

12. Jones, C. J. (1970). "Medical Ethics and Legal Questions in Human Organ Transplantation." *Journal of the National Medical Association,* 62:12–13.

13. *Hospital Tribune* (1972). "Artificial-Heart Trials Foreseen by Next Decade," 6(22):3.

14. DeBakey, M. E. (1969). "Artificial Internal Organs-I" In J. F. Dickson III, and J. H. U. Brown (eds.), *Future Goals of Engineering in Biology and Medicine.* New York: Academic Press. Pp. 172–174.

15. Landers, R. R. (1966). *Man's Place in the Dybosphere.* Englewood Cliffs, N. J.: Prentice-Hall.

16. Ferkiss, V. C. (1970). *Technological Man: The Myth and the Reality.* New York: New American Library.

17. Fletcher, J. (1974). *The Ethics of Genetic Control: Ending Reproductive Roulette.* Garden City, N. J.: Anchor.

18. Schroeder, L. O. (1974). "New Life: Person or Property?" *American Journal of Psychiatry,* 131:541–544.

19. Ramsey, P. (1970). *Fabricated Man: The Ethics of Genetic Control.* New Haven: Yale University Press.

20. Edwards, R. G. (1972). "Aspects of Human Reproduction." In W. Fuller (ed.), *The Biological Revolution: Social Good or Social Evil?* Garden City, N.J.: Doubleday. Pp. 128–142.

21. Lappé, M. (1972). "Risk-Taking for the Unborn." *Hastings Center Report,* 2(1):1–3.

22. Idant Corporation. *Considering A Vasectomy? Consider Sperm Banking First.* New York. Pamphlet.

23. *The Futurist* (1972). "Frozen Sperm Banks Will Assure 'Reversible' Vasectomies," 6(5):180.

24. Lasch, C. (1972). "Birth, Death and Technology: The Limits of Cultural Laissez-Faire." *Hastings Center Report,* 2(3):1–4.

25. *Medical World News* (1973). "Human Genetic Engineering." 14(19):45–57.

26. Lappé, M. (1973). "How Much Do We Want to Know About the Unborn?" *Hastings Center Report,* 3(1):8–9.

27. Hilton, B. (1972). "Will the Baby Be Normal? . . . And What Is the Cost of Knowing?" *Hastings Center Report,* 2(3):8–9.

28. Murray, R. F. (1974). "Genetic Disease and Human Health." *Hastings Center Report,* 4(4):4–6.

29. Lappé, M. (1973). "Genetic Knowledge and the Concept of Health." *Hastings Center Report*, 3(4):1–3.

30. Ramsay, P. (1966). "Moral and Religious Implications of Genetic Control." In J. D. Roslansky (ed.), *Genetics and the Future of Man*. New York: Appleton-Century-Crofts. Pp. 109–169.

31. Lederberg, J. (1966). "Experimental Genetics and Human Evolution." *Bulletin of the Atomic Scientists*, 22(8):4–11.

32. Penrose, L. S. (1972). "Ethics and Eugenics." In W. Fuller (ed.), *The Biological Revolution: Social Good or Social Evil?*" Garden City, N. J.: Doubleday. Pp. 112–118.

33. Beale, G. (1972). "Social Effects of Research in Human Genetics." In W. Fuller (ed.), *The Biological Revolution: Social Good or Social Evil?* Garden City, N. J.: Doubleday. Pp. 101–110.

34. Tatum. E. L. (1966). "The Possibility of Manipulating Genetic Change." In J. D. Roslansky (ed.), *Genetics and the Future of Man*. New York: Appleton-Century-Crofts. Pp. 51–61.

35. Pollock, M. R. (1972). "Molecular Genetics: Short-Term Applications and Long-Term Possibilities." In W. Fuller (ed.), *The Biological Revolution: Social Good or Social Evil?* Garden City, N. J.: Doubleday. Pp. 70–94.

36. Strauss, M. B. (ed.) (1968). *Familiar Medical Quotations*. Boston: Little, Brown.

37. Muller, H. J. (1968). "What Genetic Course Will Man Steer?" *Bulletin of the Atomic Scientists*, 24(3):6–12.

38. Davis, K. (1966). "Sociological Aspects of Genetic Control." In J. D. Roslansky (ed.), *Genetics and the Future of Man*. New York: Appleton-Century-Crofts. Pp. 173–204.

39. London, P. (1969). *Behavior Control*. New York: Harper & Row.

40. Halleck, S. L. (1974). "Legal and Ethical Aspects of Behavior Control." *American Journal of Psychiatry*, 131:381–385.

41. Steinfels, P. (1972). "Confronting the Other Drug Problem." *Hastings Center Report*, 2(5):4–6.

42. London, P. (1972). "Personal Liberty and Behavior Control Technology." *Hastings Center Report*, 2(1):4–7.

43. Michels, R. (1973). "Ethical Issues of Psychological and Psychotherapeutic Means of Behavior Control." *Hastings Center Report*, 3(2):11–13.

44. Maxmen, J. S., G. J. Tucker, and M. D. LeBow (1974). *Rational Hospital Psychiatry: The Reactive Environment*. New York: Brunner/Mazel.

45. Fisher, S. (1969). "*Primum non Nocere*: Too Much of A Good Thing?" *Seminars in Psychiatry*, 1:432–442.

46. Skinner, B. F. (1972). *Beyond Freedom and Dignity*. Toronto: Bantam.

47. Mark, V. H. (1973). "Brain Surgery in Aggressive Epileptics." *Hastings Center Report*, 3(1):1–5.

48. Livingston, K. E. (1969). "The Frontal Lobes Revisited: The Case for A Second Look." *Archives of Neurology*, 20:90–95.

49. Brown, B. S., L. A. Wienckowski, and L. W. Bivens (1973). "Psychosurgery: Perspective on A Current Issue." Bethesda, Md.: National Institute of Mental Health.

50. Baker, E. F. W., M. P. Young, D. M. Gauld, and J. F. R. Fleming (1970). "A New Look at Bimedial Prefrontal Leukotomy." *Canadian Medical Association Journal*, 102:37–41.

51. Sykes, M. K., and R. F. Tredgold (1964). "Restricted Orbital Undercutting: A Study of its Effects on 350 Patients Over the Ten Years 1951–1960." *British Journal of Psychiatry*, 110:609–640.

52. Sweet, W. H. (1973). "Treatment of Medically Intractable Mental Disease by Limited Frontal Leucotomy—Justifiable?" *New England Journal of Medicine*, 289:1117–1125.

53. Breggin, P. R. (1972). "New Information in the Debate over Psychosurgery." Congressional Record: Proceedings and Debates of the 92nd Congress, Second Session. March 30.

54. Delgado, J. M. R. (1969). *Physical Control of the Mind: Toward A Psycho-Civilized Society*. New York: Harper Colophon Books.

55. *Footnotes to the Future* (1974). "Medical Notes: Brain Pacemaker," 4(3):4.

56. Gabor, D. (1970). *Innovations: Scientific, Technological, and Social*. New York: Oxford University Press.

57. Krech, D. (1967). "Psychochemical Manipulation and Social Policy." *Annals of Internal Medicine*, 67(3) Part II, Supplement 7:19–24.

58. Milgram, S. (1974). *Obedience to Authority: An Experimental View*. New York: Harper & Row.

59. Erikson, E. H. (1974). *Dimensions of A New Identity: The 1973 Jefferson Lectures in the Humanities*. New York: Norton.

60. *The Futurist* (1973). "Ahead of Time: Some of Today's Far-Out Ideas." 7(3):130–133.

61. B. S. Eisenberg and P. Aherne (eds.) (1974). *Socioeconomic Issues of Health '74*. Chicago: American Medical Association.

62. Ettinger, R. C. W. (1969). *The Prospect of Immortality*. New York: Mac-Fadden-Bartell.

63. Prehoda, R. H. (1969). *Suspended Animation: The Research Possibility That May Allow Man to Conquer the Limiting Chains of Time*. Philadelphia: Chilton.

64. Gardner, J. W. (1972). "Uncritical Lovers, Unloving Critics." In R. Theobald (ed.), *Futures Conditional*. Indianapolis: Bobbs-Merrill. Pp. 142–148.

65. Wren-Lewis, J. (1974). "Educating Scientists for Tomorrow." In A. Toffler (ed.), *Learning For Tomorrow: The Role of the Future in Education*. New York: Vintage. Pp. 157–172.

66. Feinberg, G. (1971). "Long-Range Goals and the Environment." *The Futurist*, 5:241–246.

67. Tunney, J. V., and M. E. Levine (1972). "Genetic Engineering." *Saturday Review*, 55(32):23–28.

68. DeNike, L. D. (1972). "The Dangers of Dire Predictions." *The Futurist*, 6:118–120.

69. Roszak, T. (1968). *The Making of the Counter Culture: Reflections on the Technocratic Society and Its Youthful Opposition*. Garden City, N. J.: Doubleday.

70. Kass, L. R. (1972). *Making Babies—The New Biology and the "Old" Morality*. Hastings-on-Hudson, N. Y.: Institute of Society, Ethics and the Life Sciences.

71. Watson, J. D. (1970). "The Future of Asexual Reproduction." *Intellectual Digest*, 1(2):69–74.

72. Culliton, B. J. (1974). "National Research Act: Restores Training, Bans Fetal Research." *Hastings Center Report*, 4(4):12–13.

73. Toffler, A. (1971). *Future Shock*. New York: Bantam.

74. Taviss, I. (1971). "Problems in the Social Control of Biomedical Science and Technology." In E. Mendelsohn, J. P. Swazey, and I. Taviss (eds.), *Human Aspects of Biomedical Innovation*. Cambridge: Harvard University Press. Pp. 3–45.

75. Burger, W. E. (1967). "The Law and Medical Advances." *Annals of Internal Medicine*, 67(3) Part II, Supplement 7:15–18.

76. Babbie, E. R. (1970). *Science and Morality in Medicine: A Survey of Medical Educators*. Berkeley: University of California Press.

77. Gordon, T. J., and R. H. Ament (1969). *Forecasts of Some Technological and Scientific Developments and Their Societal Consequences*. Middletown, Conn.: Institute for the Future. Number R–6.

78. Wiener, N. (1971). *The Human Use of Human Beings: Cybernetics and Society*. New York: Avon.

7

THE ACADEME
OF TOMORROW _____

So interrelated are medicine and medical education that projecting the future of one necessitates predicting the future of the other. Not only does the nature of clinical practice influence the training of health care personnel, but the training of health care personnel inevitably alters the nature of clinical practice. Any exploration of medicine's future should entail an examination of anticipated developments in health education.

Unfortunately, the difficulties previously enumerated in forecasting the future of medicine apply equally to predicting the future of medical education. Dr. C. Sydney Burwell once observed, "My students are dismayed when I say to them, 'Half of what you are taught as medical students will in ten years have been shown to be wrong, and the trouble is, none of your teachers knows which half' " (1, p. 115). Nevertheless, we must speculate about the medical academe of tomorrow, if we are to influence how it eventually could and should materialize.

In a Post-Physician Era the training of health care personnel

will not be limited to the education of medics. Others, such as
nurses, public health officials, researchers, and administrators,
will continue to require training. I explore these topics in this
chapter and discuss medical libraries which I believe will play an
even greater role in the future training of health care professionals. At the end of this chapter I make several observations about
the future health education of the general public.

MEDICAL SCHOOLS.   Just as physicians are at the center of
the present health care delivery system, so too are medical
schools at the center of the present health care educational
system. We spend more money annually per pupil to train medical
students than we do to educate any other health care professional (2). Teaching traditionally has been an obligation of the
medical profession. The Hippocratic Oath states, ". . . by precept,
lecture and every other mode of instruction, I will impart a
knowledge of the art to my sons . . ." Thus, the importance of
training student-physicians has existed throughout medical
history. However, as we enter a Post-Physician Era, the traditional
function of the medical school will change from training doctors
to training medics. This transformation will alter how students are
admitted and what they are taught.

Although there are exceptions, a standard career path is
followed by most physicians-in-training. After graduating from
a liberal arts college, a student is accepted by a medical school
primarily on the basis of his scientific proficiencies. As Dr.
William Bradford notes, "All medical school catalogues extol the
virtues of the broad liberal arts education, but when the chips
are down, only the applicants with top grades in science get in,
and the students know it" (3, p. 57). Generally, medical students
embark upon a four year program. The basic medical sciences
are emphasized during the first two years to convey an understanding of fundamental health and disease concepts. The
student is introduced to clinical medicine during the last two
years. Upon graduation, the novice physician usually acquires
two to four years of additional training which prepares him to

practice in a particular specialty area, such as pediatrics, surgery, psychiatry, and so on.

In a Post-Physician Era this process will change significantly. Because the computer will render the vast majority of diagnostic and treatment decisions, the medic will not have to possess a basic understanding of health and disease concepts. Because medics will not need to learn chemistry, biology, physics, etc., they will not have to graduate from a liberal arts college to be eligible for medical school. Interpersonal talents will replace scientific sophistication as the major admission criterion. Prior experience working with people would be a strongly desired or even mandatory requirement. Although personal interviews of candidates are conducted at most contemporary medical schools, they generally are not very influential in determining who will be admitted. In a Post-Physician Era personal interviews will be more significant. They could be held in person or conducted via interactive television or phonovision. In addition, although none currently exist, by the outset of the 21st century psychological tests may provide accurate measurements of an applicant's actual or potential interpersonal abilities.

A doctor's training lasts approximately eight years; the standard education for a medic will be 12 to 18 months. The feasibility of successfully training medics during this relatively brief period will depend primarily upon the selection of individuals who possess certain personality characteristics. More specifically, they would have to be able to empathize with, be sensitive to, and be tolerant of people with physical and emotional disorders. They should be sufficiently introspective and psychologically mature to identify and control their own feelings. They must be honest, dependable, efficient, thorough, energetic, and intelligent. In my experience as a psychiatric educator I have found that no amount of training can embue someone with these personality characteristics. To be an effective practitioner from an interpersonal standpoint, an applicant must have acquired these qualities *prior* to entering medical school. Training can enable a student to develop and refine his innate abilities, but it cannot inculcate him with basic talents he never had. To take anybody

off the street and expect him to function properly as a medic
would be a plan doomed to failure. Thus the most critical prerequisite for successfully training medics in only 12 to 18 months
is selecting individuals who already have the necessary personality characteristics.

Once people with these qualities have been chosen, their
medical school training could expand upon and channel their
innate abilities so that they could provide supportive patient care.
Despite the many subjects that student medics would need to
learn, there already is evidence that people who previously have
the aforementioned characteristics could be trained in 12 to 18
months. For example, at the Bronx Municipal Hospital Center,
psychiatric rehabilitation workers (PRWs) have been taught to
conduct individual and family psychotherapy as well as to perform
social service and team leadership functions. Because they have
been selected carefully, possess the qualities previously enumerated, and have been trained effectively, they practice their skills
with a high degree of reliability, dedication, and sophistication.
The talents required of PRWs are similar to those that will be
needed by medics. Most relevant to this discussion, however, is
the fact that these PRWs are trained in only *one year*. As new
educational techniques develop, our ability to train medics even
more effectively and efficiently should increase.

The 12 to 18 months of concentrated training medics would
receive in providing supportive care would be almost 12 to 18
months more instruction than is currently obtained by doctors.
Student-physicians who establish excellent patient rapport are
able to do so in large measure because of the interpersonal abilities
they had prior to entering medical school, even with little, if any,
instruction in developing and maintaining an effective doctor-
patient relationship. Because medics would not have to learn an
extensive amount of technical information, most of their training
could focus upon the delivery of supportive care. And just as the
student-physician's education does not end when he graduates,
the medic also would be expected to continue learning once he is
in practice.

Once admitted to medical school, the first half of the medic's education would be primarily didactic, while the second half would be primarily clinical. Upon graduation, the medic would have the option of functioning as a generalist or as a specialist. If he chose the latter course, he would require further training to learn about conducting psychotherapy, delivering babies, setting fractures, and so on. Other medics may decide to enter administration or education.

The overall objective of the student's medical school education would be to prepare him to function within a medic-computer model. To accomplish this goal the curriculum would have to focus upon the following areas: the psychology of illness, family dynamics, group processes, medical sociology, medical terminology, medical ethics, patient administration, and the technology of supportive care.

The Psychology of Illness.   The student would need to be aware of the many ways that patients react to and cope with disease. Kahana and Bibring have outlined seven personality tyeps and attitudes frequently encountered by practitioners. These are the dependent, overdemanding personality; the orderly, controlled personality; the dramatizing, emotionally involved, captivating personality; the long-suffering, self-sacrificing individual; the guarded, querulous, suspicious patient; the person with excessive feelings of superiority; and the patient who appears uninvolved and aloof (4). In addition to learning how to identify these personality characteristics, student-medics also would need to appreciate the psychological meaning of an illness to a patient and that this meaning could vary from individual to individual. For example, to one person the diagnosis of ulcers may signify that he has failed to cope with the stresses of life, while to another person the same diagnosis would arouse irrational fears of imminent death. In attempting to learn the personal meaning of illness to patients, the student-medic would have to be aware of his own feelings toward disease so that he would not mistakenly ascribe those feelings to his patients.

Family Dynamics.   Because the meaning of an illness and the way in which a patient deals with it can be affected significantly by the important people in a patient's environment, the student-medic should learn some fundamental principles of family dynamics. A knowledge of both the overt and the more subtle ways in which relatives influence the patient's attempts to cope with his disease would be helpful. For example, I once treated a 17-year-old boy who was hospitalized repeatedly for diabetic coma. Initially, his mother appeared to be a responsible parent who was very concerned about her son's health, but further investigation revealed that since the patient's father had died from a stroke five years before, the mother had invested all her emotional energies in her son. Because the boy was an only child, the mother was afraid that he would soon go away to college and leave her alone. She also worried that unless her son had sufficient exercise, he, like his father, would become enfeebled or even die from a stroke. Consequently, she pushed her son into highly competitive athletics, claiming that she did not want her "child to become an invalid because of the diabetes." She told me that despite her repeated encouragement she could not understand why her son often refused to take his insulin; the more she protested the more recalcitrant her son became. The combination of excessive exercise and failure to take medication resulted in his numerous hospitalizations. Her actions seriously aggravated the son's illness so that he would be unable to attend college and would have to remain at home as a companion and surrogate husband for this superficially reasonable, but covertly overprotective, parent. For a medic to implement effectively the treatment decisions of the computer, he would have to identify family interactional patterns. He should also clarify and understand his feelings toward his own family so that he would not falsely ascribe motives and behavior to the relatives of his patients.

Group Processes.   To attend optimally to the supportive needs of his patients and their families and to participate constructively as a member of the health care team, medics would need to become sensitive to group processes. The understanding of authority relationships, leadership struggles, resistances to change and cooperation are a few of the issues that would enhance the medic's performance.

Medical Sociology. The effect that culture plays in a patient's apperception of disease and treatment should occupy a prominent position in the medical school's curriculum. The acquisition of a sociological perspective would supplement the medic's understanding of his patient's reactions to illness. For example, one study in a New York hospital revealed that Italians and Jews had differing concerns about pain. Italian patients wanted relief from pain and were reasonably satisfied when this relief was obtained; Jewish subjects were primarily worried about the meaning and significance of the pain and its potential consequences for the future (5). Although these findings obviously represent generalizations, they do underscore the importance of an awareness that different economic, cultural, and racial groups often have divergent concerns about illness and varying expectations from treatment.

Medical Terminology. Although a medic's training will be directed primarily toward enhancing his interpersonal skills, he still will require an elementary knowledge of medical terminology to relate the computer's findings and recommendations to his patients.

Medical Ethics. As outlined in the previous chapter, biomedical innovations will present society with many new ethical dilemmas. I argued in that chapter that the major responsibility for contending with these ethical issues must fall upon the individual. In the future patients are going to have to decide whether they will utilize a controversial technique, such as artificial insemination, genetic manipulation, and cryogenic preservation. If a medic is to help his patients in reaching a decision, he must be aware of not only the potential psychological impact that such a decision could exert, but also the ethical problems that ought to be considered before finalizing that decision. The medic will need to identify his own ethical standards and learn how to avoid imposing these values on his clients. Training in medical ethics should impart to the medic an understanding of what constitutes ethical clinical practice. Maintaining confidentiality, respecting patient dignity, assuming appropriate responsibility, placing the needs of patients above one's own are all ideals to be inculcated throughout the medic's education.

Patient Administration. The medic will have to become thoroughly familiar with the varying administrative procedures that will be established in a Post-Physician Era. He also will need to know how to operate medical computers to obtain their diagnostic decisions and treatment recommendations. Because some patients may have difficulties or be unable to give their histories to a computer, the medic will have to acquire skills in assisting patients to interact with the machine. Of course by the advent of a Post-Physician Era the ability to operate medical computers would be a relatively simple skill to acquire because automation will be utilized widely throughout society.

The Technology of Supportive Care. All of the seven previous subject areas should be taught with the aim of providing the medic with a foundation upon which he will be able to offer patients high-quality supportive care. Many of the complaints registered against contemporary doctors are that they fail to meet the emotional and educative needs of their patients (6–8). Physicians speak about the "art and science" of medicine. The "art" refers to the provision of supportive care, and the "science" pertains to the performance of technical services. This distinction is illuminating in that it implies that whereas the science of medicine can be taught, the art of medicine cannot. Most medical school faculty act as if the ability to relate to patients is innate and that no amount of training can significantly enhance this skill. Although many professors may disavow this belief, I maintain that it is a widely prevalent one, because very few contemporary medical schools systematically train students in the technology of supportive care. Furthermore, I would suggest that the lack of such training does *not* occur because a technology of supportive care is unavailable;* it occurs because the need to absorb the science of medicine becomes an overriding and, for the most part, a legitimate educational priority for reasons enumerated in Chapter 2. Training in the technology of supportive care is a minimal, if not an altogether missing, part of modern-day medical curricula.

In contrast to a physician-centered model, under a medic-computer system, teaching the technology of supportive care would be the primary educational endeavor. Although a comprehensive discussion of how this task could be accomplished is beyond the scope of this book, several potential techniques and approaches are worth noting. In making these comments I wish to emphasize that there are two aspects of the topic to be considered—the technology of *giving* supportive care and the technology of *training* people to give supportive care.

In an attempt to study doctor-patient communication Korsch and Neguete tape recorded 800 sessions in which a mother, her sick child, and a pediatrician conversed during a clinic visit. After the session one of the investigators interviewed the mother to solicit her reactions to the visit. Although there were other aspects of the study, this part of the investigation revealed the following: There was no significant correlation between the length of a patient's visit and the mother's satisfaction with the encounter. The investigators noted that some of the longest sessions were spent not with performing diagnostic activities, but with attempting to understand what the other person was saying.

The study also showed that more than half of the physicians utilized too much technical language in talking with the mothers.

* Indeed many books deal with this subject (9–11).

Although some mothers were impressed, if not flattered, by the use of medical jargon, it often resulted in the mothers being confused and unenlightened about the nature of their children's illnesses. For example, the authors found that one mother thought a "lumbar puncture" meant to drain the lungs, while another did not realize that to "explore" referred to surgery. Another observation was that less than 5 percent of the physician's conversation was personal or friendly. Not only did many of the parents feel that the pediatrician did not care about them or their children, but frequently the doctors blamed the mothers for causing their child's disease. One physician even said, "Stevie, it's your mother's fault that you have this high fever." Although the comment may have been made in jest, the mother later expressed great distress over the remark.

A common source of dismay for these mothers was that the doctor revealed a total disregard for what concerned them. For example, when one parent repeatedly tried to interest the pediatrician in her child's vomiting, she felt the doctor was ignoring her because he only asked about other symptoms, such as dehydration. Although the physician knew that there was a direct relationship between dehydration and vomiting, the mother did not. Because the doctor failed to explain this connection or even to recognize the mother's frustration, the visit ended without a positive rapport ever being established. Very often this breakdown in communication led to so much hostility on the part of the mother that she was unable to hear the information and advice that actually was given to her by the physician. In about 20 percent of the cases the doctor failed to tell the parent what was wrong with the child. And finally, tape recordings of the sessions revealed that doctors did more talking than mothers and that when this occurred, parental satisfaction declined (7).

Among other reasons, this study is significant because it specifically identifies how physician-patient communication can go astray. The authors noted that in discussing their findings with the involved pediatricians, most of them were unaware of their excessive use of technical language, their failure to respond to the mothers' concerns, and so on (7). I would suggest that the breakdowns in communication resulted not because the doctors were malevolent, but because they were oblivious to and untrained in effective communication skills. This difficulty could be overcome by using several techniques. After a clinic visit student-medics could receive direct feedback from the patient regarding the nature of the interview. Another approach would be to videotape sessions and subsequently analyze the recordings. Videotapes have been utilized extensively in the training of psychotherapists (12–14); they also have been used to sensitize contemporary student physicians to their relationships with medical patients.

Harvard internists, psychiatrists, and students have collaborativley discussed trainee-conducted interviews. They have focused upon six general areas: medical diagnosis and treatment, interviewing and communication techniques, psychological characteristics of the patient, the use of the doctor-patient relationship, the inter-disciplinary care of the patient, and psychosocial aspects of illness. Both faculty and students have responded favorably to these exercises (15). Videotaping clinical interviews not only allows the trainee to focus upon these six areas, but it also permits them to assess nonverbal behavior which is being increasingly recognized as a significant aspect of communication (16–17). The greater availability and the decreasing costs of portable videotape equipment (18) suggests that the use of these devices may have a more prominent place in the technological armamentarium of future medical educators. The opportunity to teach systematically the effective use of communication skills will be available under a medic-computer model.

The use of sensitivity groups could play a major role in medic education. Participating in such an experience may afford students an opportunity to enhance their understanding of group processes; sharpen their sensitivity to the psychological nuances of interpersonal relations; and help them become more aware of their own feelings, attitudes, and behaviors. As long as these groups limit their focus to these areas, instead of attempting to provide psychotherapy, experiences with contemporary medical students who have participated in these groups demonstrate that they can be highly successful (19). Other types of group encounters also may be beneficial. Meetings between student-medics and patients that would concentrate on relationships between health care professionals and consumers may help to sensitize students to the concerns of patients, while informing patients about the problems faced by medics.

Because both the theoretical training and the practical clinical experience of the medic will necessitate interdisciplinary cooperation, discussion groups with medics, technical nurses, social workers, computer experts, and other health care professionals may prove to be a worthwhile experience. During their psychiatric clerkship, Dartmouth medical and nursing students had conjoint sessions in which they exchanged views about the problems each discipline had working with the other. The nursing students echoed Florence Nightingale's sentiment, "It seems a commonly received idea among men and even among women themselves that it requires nothing but a disappointment in love, the want of an object, a general disgust, or an incapacity for other things, to turn a woman into a good nurse" (20, p. 322). Nursing students resented the condescending attitude of doctors and the latter's reluctance to involve them in clinical and educational experiences. They also acknowledged their own unrealistic expectations of physicians as well as their tendency to forget that medical house staff, like themselves, are frequently scrutinized and pressured by their superiors. Student-physicians objected to the passivity and immaturity of many nurses as well as to their own proclivity to ignore nurses or treat them as glorified maids. These provocative meetings were highly successful, and some of the participants felt they were the highlight of their entire academic careers. Because these seminars were of only brief duration, they probably did not have any lasting influence upon the participants. Nevertheless, if these meetings could be held *throughout* their training, they possibly could have an enduring effect. One could hypothesize that in a Post-Physician Era these interdisciplinary sensitivity groups could be a valuable part of a medic's curriculum.

The technology of supportive care may be enhanced by the more extensive use of behavior modification. In recent years there have been many claims that behavior modification is a cruel and sadistic form of treatment. Films, such as *The Clockwork Orange*, and even the writings of prominent mental health professionals, such as Seymour Halleck (21), argue that behavior modification is a dehumanizing approach to patient care. For the most part these charges have been unfounded. Of course, there are occasions when behavior therapists have deployed electric shocks or deprived people of food or other vital necessities to produce adaptive change. However, these practices are the exception and not the rule. Most experienced behaviorists would deplore the use of these drastic measures because they recognize that in these instances the treatment is worse than the disease. Moreover, they would maintain that if the practitioner has to resort to these dehumanizing techniques, something is awry with the behavioral program being employed (22). Like any other method in medicine, behavior modification can be used to the patient's benefit or to his detriment. Despite the lurid images often evoked by the phrase *behavior modification*, the fact is that modifying behavior is an unavoidable and necessary aspect of the interaction between a healer and his patient. The critical question is not if we should use behavior modification, but rather how it should be done to enhance the patient's sense of well-being.

To discuss the wide repertoire of behavior modification techniques in the practice of medicine would be beyond the scope of this book. Furthermore, for the reader to understand how these methods could be employed clinically, he would have to possess a fundamental understanding of behavioral principles—a subject that also would be too extensive to cover in this chapter. Nevertheless, at the risk of being overly simplistic, I will give one example of an application of a behavioral technique to convey a sense of how these methods could be employed by medics in the provision of patient care.

Patients with chronic pain present numerous difficulties to physicians, nurses, and relatives. Very often the cries of anguish from these patients is out of proportion to the amount of pain they are actually experiencing. Being totally bedridden, they can be found whining, grimacing, and demanding the affection and care of others. Under usual circumstances, whenever these patients complain about their symptoms they receive a great amount of attention and are often given ever-increasing doses of narcotics. Not only do these patients frequently become addicted, they often alienate everybody around them because of their constant moaning. In analyzing these problems a behaviorist may observe that giving attention and dispensing medication whenever the patient complains of pain reinforces or encourages the patient to continue his complaining. Therefore, attempts to make the patient more comfortable often have the paradoxical effect of aggravating his symptoms. One study showed that this problem can be overcome by changing the patterns of reinforcement. Patients with chronic pain were given narcotics at regular intervals rather than when they fretted about their pain. They received attention only when they were *not* complaining of pain and were engaged in constructive activities. The use of medication and the granting of attention were not contingent upon the patients' cries of discomfort. Instead, the drugs and attention were utilized to promote the exhibition of adaptive behaviors. By using this technique, narcotic dosages could be reduced and patients could live more gratifying existences while experiencing considerably less pain than before the behavioral program was instituted (23).*

In a Post-Physician Era student-medics could be trained in the clinical application of behavior modification. They would learn to execute behavioral protocols that would help patients to take their medication, to control their weight, and to exercise properly. Instead of resorting to tranquilizers, patients could be taught systematic relaxation methods as a way of coping with anxiety.

Training medics in behavior modification also would have the benefit of enhancing their ability to identify environmental stresses that might trigger physical symptoms. Fundamental to behaviorism is the notion that human activity is almost, if not totally, a response to environmental forces. Behaviorists maintain

* In practice, the use of this technique is more complicated than I have presented it. However, for the sake of simplicity and space I have only touched upon the highlights of the program. A more detailed discussion of the use of behavior modification in medical practice can be found elsewhere (10).

that by identifying all of the variables influencing an organism, one can predict how a person will act and that by altering these variables behavioral change can occur (10, 24). Although many people do not accept these behavioral premises, few individuals would deny the overwhelming influence environmental events exert upon human behavior.

The current use of behavioral technology has been limited in that we are often unable to identify the significant variables influencing behavior. Once we are able to identify the critical determinants of a particular behavior, we will probably find that they consist of a great number of parameters with very complex interrelationships. The computer might be necessary to predict how the alteration of these variables would modify the patient's activities. Already machines have been used successfully to forecast how government narcotic policies would alter addiction and crime rates. These predictions were made by isolating the critical social forces and human responses and running them through a computer analysis (25). Similarly, medics could use the machine to identify the critical determinants of a patient's behavior. Then they could use the computer to discover how environmental forces could be modified to promote the desired behavioral response or to deter the occurrence of distressing symptomatology.

The principles and techniques of behavior modification also could be used in training medics. For example, I noted earlier that teaching communication skills will be important if medics are to become proficient in the technology of supportive care. However, teaching a skill to a student is quite different from having him routinely and properly implement it. In the future we might be able to discover better methods for reinforcing the performance of effective communication skills by medics and other health care professionals. Behavioral techniques that encourage the execution of other supportive care activities also could be devised and utilized as a routine part of a medic's training (22).

Another important task faced by the medic in providing supportive care will be the need to offer patients information about their illnesses. Because medics will not have a sufficient knowledge of diseases and their treatment, they will have to rely upon computers to acquire this information. Later in this chapter I discuss Health Science Information Centers, which will be the medical libraries of the future. For now, however, I wish only to note that these institutions will be able to provide medics with instantaneous answers to any questions patients may have about their condition. Medics will have to be trained to obtain this information and learn effective means of conveying it to their patients.

In addition to the many learning techniques already enumerated, medics will be taught the principles and technology of supportive care by both traditional educational mediums (e.g., books, lectures, small-group discussions) and by newer automated teaching devices such as computer-aided instruction (CAI) (26–27) and computer-aided simulation (CAS) (28–33). Already these technological teachers are gaining popularity among medical educators. In the fall of 1972 a survey of 801 health science schools revealed that of the 561 that responded, 78 reported that their schools were using some kind of computerized teaching systems, and an additional 116 expected to do so in the near future. This study also showed that automated learning devices most frequently were employed in medical schools to teach clinical subjects. The Ohio State University College of Medicine developed 44 percent of the programs, while 74 percent came from only three institutions. This survey suggests that despite their relative novelty, computerized teaching methods have gained a moderate amount of acceptance, and their use may increase in the future, especially as remote access to these programs becomes available via the experimental communications network of the National Library of Medicine's Lister Hill National Center for Biomedical Communications (34).

As medical schools are transformed from institutions to train physicians in the technical aspects of clinical medicine into facilities to equip medics with the ability to provide the technology of supportive care, they also will be undergoing other organizational modifications. One of the most important alterations may be in the relationship between medical schools and other health care training institutions. For example, at present most medical, public health, and nursing schools function autonomously, each with their own students, curriculum, administration, faculty, and so on. Although this organizational structure inhibits the establishment of interdisciplinary programs (35–36), as long as a physician-centered model persists, this suboptimal arrangement may not create any *major* difficulties. Because a health-team and a medic-computer model would necessitate closer working relationships between professionals, the rigid boundaries that currently exist between health care training facilities will have to be reduced substantially. Medical progress is becoming increasingly dependent upon contributions from disciplines, such as engineering, mathematics, and sociology, that traditionally have not been adequately represented within health care training facilities (36). If educational programs are to capitalize fully upon their resources, structural reorganization of existing training institutions may be required.

COLLEGE OF HEALTH SCIENCES. The need to integrate or at least to coordinate training programs could be enhanced by the creation of Colleges of Health Sciences (CHS). These colleges may consist of six major educational institutions: medical schools, nursing schools, health science information centers, schools of medical management, public health schools, and schools of medical investigation. The following comments are intended to suggest some general principles under which a CHS and its constituent schools potentially could operate.

The *raison d'être* of establishing a College of Health Sciences would be to maximize cooperation between its member schools. A CHS would be pointless unless it would facilitate interdisciplinary programs and minimize institutional boundaries. Although these goals are widely accepted in principle, at present there is no coordinating body among most contemporary health care training institutions with either the responsibility or the authority to implement them. To be effective, the leadership of a CHS would have to be entrusted with this power. It could include representatives from each of the health science schools, headed by a chairman or a dean who would function as a creative synthetic executive. The tasks of this coordinating body can be divided somewhat arbitrarily into intramural and extramural activities.

One of its intramural responsibilities would be to set financial priorities, while ensuring that each of its constituent schools would receive an equitable share of the funds. It also would help students of one school to enter courses in another school. For example, at present a student nurse who wishes to take a class from experts in managerial techniques finds enrollment in a hospital administration course almost impossible. Every time a student wishes to do such a thing extensive negotiations between the hierarchies of each school are required. The leadership of a CHS would be in the position to implement interschool student exchanges.

A CHS also could establish new courses for all health science students. Presently, within the same medical complex schools of medicine, nursing, and public health may all have their own class in, for example, statistics. A CHS could eliminate this duplication by offering a *single* statistics course. This coordinated effort would be economically advantageous and would foster contact between occupational groups. The leadership of a CHS could employ individuals whose specific and unusual areas of expertise would preclude them from being full-time members of any one school. For instance, although a nursing school could benefit from the services of a communications technologist, it may either be unable to afford one on a full-time basis or only need their skills to a limited extent. A CHS could hire such an expert as a consultant-at-large to assist students and faculty in every school.

In the 19th century most physicians practiced medicine without any appreciable understanding of basic health and disease processes. The Flexner revolution of 1911 rectified this deficiency by guaranteeing that doctors would acquire a solid foundation in the basic sciences and be trained within approved hospital settings (37). As a result, most medical schools were built adjacent to hospitals. An unfortunate consequence was that medical schools became increasingly separated, both geographically and intellectually, from the main campuses of universities. As Irving London has observed, "For many years, the improvements in medical education engendered by the Flexner report obscured the disadvantages that derived from such intellectual isolation. But in recent years, these disadvantages have become more obvious" (35, p. 43). Noting the importance of computer science, anthropology, physics, psychology, systems analysis, and so on, London states, "Indeed, one may fairly argue that the wide gap that exists between the potential of the medical sciences and the actuality of health care derives in part from the insular relationships of medical education to these other sciences and disciplines" (35, p. 44). The primary extramural task of a CHS should be to forge a closer alliance with the university (35–36). By making this relationship a bidirectional one, both the university and the CHS would profit. Physical anthropology students could take anatomy courses in schools of medical investigation, and future hospital administrators could avail themselves of sociology classes. The leadership of a CHS could import, for example, law professors to serve periodically as consultants to any or all of the health care schools.

Although many contemporary health care training institutions are associated with universities, this affiliation usually exists in name only. For example, although medical schools are nominally a part of the university's organization, they are generally not a part of the university's budget. The prevailing notion is that because medical schools can be reimbursed for providing patient services, they ought to be economically self-sufficient (38). This fiscal arrangement tends to isolate the medical school from its parent university. Although the latter feels justified in supporting basic research and teaching within its own liberal arts college, it feels little obligation to support similar activities within its own medical school. If health care training institutions are to become a more integral part of universities, their relationship must be a fiscal as well as a structural one.

There are two other important extramural functions for a

CHS. The first is the responsibility to acquire financial support from private and government agencies. Currently, nursing, medical, and public health schools often fail to cooperate and at times even compete among themselves to raise funds. The existence of CHSs could overcome these difficulties by coordinating and unifying their fund-raising activities. The last major extramural task of a CHS would be to establish effective relations with and be accountable to the general community. The leadership of a CHS and each of its constituent schools may wish to include members from the general community. Failure to do so may risk isolating health care training institutions from the people they ultimately are intended to serve.

Because health educational facilities are dependent largely upon government funding (38), financial incentives from all levels of government may be necessary in order to create Colleges of Health Sciences to accomplish these intramural and extramural objectives.

Schools of Medical Management. Training health care administrators would be the responsibility of schools of medical management. They also could provide courses for other health care students who wish to augment their administrative skills. This opportunity would be especially helpful for those practitioners who will be leaders of health care teams. Ombudsmen would benefit from and possibly even be required to take classes in a school of medical management. Included in its faculty could be health care planners, systems engineers, businessmen, urbanologists, architects, economists, and political scientists (35).

In Chapter 3 I indicated that the emergence of a Post-Physician Era will provide health care planners with a fresh opportunity to implement some fundamental changes in the organizational structures of the American medical system. Undoubtedly, graduates of schools of medical management could play a significant role in executing these transformations. However, their ability to make appropriate modifications may be limited if they perpetuate many of the attitudes held by present counterparts.

Contemporary administrators often view organizational change as only a technical enterprise without considering either the ideological or the psychological forces that frequently underlie organizational conflict. By maintaining this technical perspective administrators act as if efficiency is the primary goal of a health care organization. This attitude often leads them to institute rigorous controls which some critics believe inhibit creative and humanistic innovation (39). In the future administrators will have to establish organizational structures that can be quickly adapted to the accelerating rate of social and medical change. However, if administrators are preoccupied with establishing rigorous controls, then their organizational structures will lack the increased flexibility that will be needed in the New Medical Order. If schools of medical management are to graduate students that will be able to contend with these organizational challenges, their curricula will have to be addressed to the technical issues of administration as well as the ideological, political, psychological, and humanistic concerns of their day.

Public Health Schools.   Students in public health schools would be trained in food production, housing, nutrition, toxicology, environmental studies, and population control, as well as in the effects of political, social, and economic forces upon health (35). As our understanding of man's ecosystem expands, public health students will be trained to monitor the environment by using wireless telemetry, closed circuit television, on-line computers, radar, sonar, microwave, and infrared sensing devices. The information derived from these instruments may enable them to discover and rectify the biogeochemical causes of illness. They also will learn to assemble synthetic life-support systems for use on spaceships, the ocean floor, and possibly other planets (40). As the effects of overpopulation and malnutrition in other countries are felt in the United States (41–42), public health students will need to be trained to deal with these problems.

In the future these students will pursue their studies from the perspective of a positive rather than a negative definition of health. The former implies man's ability to take advantage of all his physical and mental potentialities; the latter refers to the absence of disease (40). Oriented toward this positive definition of health, students will study the psychological, social, and biological effects upon man of a rapidly changing technological society. To acquire this information public health students must draw upon the intellectual resources of the other health science schools as well as the university-at-large.

Schools of Medical Investigation (SMI). A multidisciplinary research training consortium in schools of medical investigation will be necessary because of the students they will graduate, the research they will generate, and the spirit of inquiry they could foster within an entire CHS. In his famed report Abraham Flexner wrote:

> The practitioners of modern medicine must be alert, systematic, thorough, critically open-minded; they will get no such training from perfunctory teachers. Educationally, then, research is required at the medical faculty because only research will keep the teachers in condition. A nonproductive school, conceivably up-to-date today, would be out-of-date tomorrow; its dead atmosphere would soon breathe unenlightened dogmatism (37, p. 346).

Training medical researchers is both intellectually and financially advantageous. The development of drugs to treat mental illness and tuberculosis alone yielded a savings of over $1.9 billion in 1967, a sum greater than the total investment in research during that year (36). The training of medical investigators will play a vital role in medicine's future, and the only question is how this should be accomplished.

The present system has numerous disadvantages. Within any single university complex institutional boundaries inhibit the crossfertilization of ideas. Medical researchers are trained in a wide array of graduate departments, including chemistry, sociology, biology, and engineering, as well as in medical schools. Unfortunately, the students and faculty of these departments are usually separated geographically and politically and therefore, intellectually from one another. This isolation probably retards the pace of medical progress and interferes with the development of integrated curricula in the medical sciences. Investigators who are trained in university graduate departments frequently are unable to obtain access to patients, medical school faculty, and facilities.

Ph.D. candidates who are trained within medical school departments often feel like second-class citizens. As leaders of medical schools, physicians see their major responsibility to be the education of doctors, not basic scientists. They justify this view by noting that for every 100 student-physicians enrolled in medical school there are only 21 Ph.D. graduate students. Furthermore, because clinical faculty are able to raise funds for the school by delivering patient care, they often control the budgetary purse strings. Consequently, as a "minority group," Ph.D. students frequently believe they are denied their fair share of money, space, equipment, and faculty time. Sometimes this alleged discrimination generates friction between M.D. and Ph.D. investigators which may inhibit their collaboration. Because medical school trained Ph.D.s usually are sequestered within basic science departments, they have minimal exposure to clinical problems. As a result, when conducting research many Ph.D.s have difficulty recognizing and understanding the direct relevancy of their work to human problems.

Although physician-investigators are better able to relate their experiments to clinical issues, they are poorly trained in research methodology. Investigatory techniques cannot be learned during the four years of medical school; it is hardly enough time to learn medicine. At best, medical students can spend only one summer doing research (36). Even after graduation their research training is continuously interrupted by patient care responsibilities. This discontinuity may retard their investigatory efforts and discourage them from pursuing further research.

Although the establishment of schools of medical investigation may not alleviate all of these problems, it may resolve some of them. The major purposes for centralizing medical research

within a single administrative unit would be to enhance interdisciplinary cooperation and to improve managerial and economic
efficiency. The faculty of an SMI would include teachers from
both the social and the natural sciences. SMI students could be
graduates of a liberal arts college or any of the other health science
schools. Undoubtedly, all SMI students could be required to take
a core curriculum consisting of subjects such as the philosophy of
science, research methodology, statistics, applied computer technology, and biomedical ethics. Additional seminars would be
necessary according to the student's particular area of interest.

The classes available in an SMI would vary according to the prevailing model of health care delivery. As long as doctors will need
to be trained, basic science courses (e.g. anatomy, microbiology,
physiology) may be taught and clinical science courses (e.g.
surgery, pediatrics, neurology) definitely will be taught within
medical schools.

In a Post-Physician Era, however, medics would not have to
take these courses; hence, there would be no reason for a medical
school to offer them. Nevertheless, they still would have to be
available for students who wish to pursue research on these
particular subjects. Furthermore, it was noted in Chapter 1 that
surgery will be the last function of the physician to be rendered
obsolete by a medic-computer symbiosis. Thus, within the next
50 years some surgical interventions may still be the treatment of
choice for certain diseases. Medics could easily learn to conduct
procedures that are relatively simple to perform, but operations
that involve a high degree of technical sophistication will have to
be performed by someone with extensively developed skills.
These operations may become so specialized that only an SMI
could provide an individual with the appropriate training.

Under a medic-computer model, courses in the basic and
clinical sciences that presently are taught in medical schools
would be taught in SMIs. For the most part these courses will
emphasize their methodological and investigatory aspects, rather
than focus upon their clinical applications.

In addition to educating medical researchers, an SMI also
could make selected courses available to students in other health

science schools and offer refresher classes to older investigators. In the future, as the rate of medical discoveries and innovative research techniques accelerate, it will become increasingly difficult for investigators to keep abreast of current developments. Just as continuing education is needed for today's physician, it also will be necessary for tomorrow's researcher. The final major responsibility of the faculty will be to train researchers who will be able to collect and analyze clinical data to update computer programs utilized in rendering patient care decisions. Instructing people to perform these skills will be necessary, if a medic-computer model is to become a reality.

All the schools under the administrative control of a College of Health Science will also be linked to a health science information center. This automated library of the future will be the storehouse of medical knowledge, and as such will play a critical role in the operations of tomorrow's health care academe.

HEALTH SCIENCE INFORMATION CENTERS. Traditionally, health science publications have been entombed in a literary mausoleum more commonly known as the medical library. Often bibliomanical librarians seem to view their books as museum pieces to be cherished rather than as resource materials to be utilized (43, 44). Most experts, including many librarians themselves, agree that the library has failed to achieve its primary objective—to provide relevant information both rapidly and easily (26). Medical libraries are unable to perform this function because of the rapid proliferation of professional literature. In 1967 alone the National Library of Medicine indexed almost one-quarter million articles, books, and monographs (45). The number of medical publications has been doubling every 15 years, and there is every reason to believe that this trend will continue (44). Thus, the location and retrieval of information has become progressively more difficult (43). The exponential growth of the literature, as well as the space needed to store it, is placing a progressively greater strain upon the fiscal resources of the modern medical library (46). This dilemma would be compounded further if these libraries contained the many nonmedical volumes that would be useful. Often researchers and other health science students need information from sources that, although relevant to their work, are not to be found within medical libraries. For example, books on subjects ranging from anthropology to zoology generally are unavailable in medical libraries.

By capitalizing upon recent technological developments medical libraries are gradually overcoming these problems by transforming themselves into health science information centers (HSICs). The principal objective of an HSIC is to transmit relevant information easily, quickly, and economically. Although, at least theoretically, this goal is shared by the traditional medical library, the HSIC could make it a reality. Instead of being a massive collection of books, an HSIC more closely resembles a complex audio-visual electronic laboratory.

Until recently acquiring a list of references to a particular subject was a tedious and time-consuming endeavor. However, this process was simplified considerably with the introduction of MEDLINE in 1971. If an investigator wants to review the literature on the treatment of gout, for example, he tells the librarian the key words of the subject he wishes to research. In this case they would be *gout* and *treatment*. The librarian electronically transmits these code words to the National Library of Medicine where a computer contains a list of over 400,000 articles from more than a 1000 of the world's most prominent biomedical journals. These articles are classified according to their subject, author, language, publication year, journal title, and entry date. After automatically searching its file, the machine generates and returns to the librarian all references having to do with the treatment of gout. Unless the bibliography is unusually lengthy, this can occur within a few minutes (47), and the cost is nominal. Since its inception MEDLINE has been introduced into numerous medical libraries, and eventually it may be made available to hospitals and doctor's offices (46).

One of MEDLINE's current limitations is that it only provides a list of references. Although this bibliography can be valuable, the doctor's interests may be restricted to one particular aspect of a subject. For example, a physician who receives a list of 300 references on the treatment of gout may wish to learn about the long-term efficacy of probenecid, a drug commonly used in the treatment of the disorder. Unfortunately, the title of an article often does not accurately reflect or clarify its content. The doctor may have to scurry around the library unearthing and reading 300 articles to find the few that discuss the long-range value of probenecid. This time-consuming process could be reduced if a 100-word abstract summarizing the content of each article on the list were available. It could be written by the author of the article or by a librarian. In the near future computers may be able to generate their own abstracts. In either case, these abstracts could be included with their corresponding references on the MED-LINE printout, filed in a card catalog, photographed onto microfilm, or programmed into a computer. All the user would have to do is to scan the abstracts of the articles enumerated on the MEDLINE bibliography and then retrieve only the ones that are germane to his interests. Some authorities believe that this service may become widely available before the end of this decade (46).

The problem of storing the accelerated number of journals, books, and monographs may be solved if all medical literature were microfilmed. A Bible consisting of 1245 pages with 773,746 words can be reproduced on a transparency about the size of one typical 35 mm slide. If photographed onto microfilm, 42 million pieces occupying 270 miles of shelves in the United States Library of Congress could be stored in only six standard filing cabinets. One major problem with microfilm, however, is the expense involved. To place the 42 million pieces of the United States Library of Congress onto microfilm initially would cost about $500 million. However, subsequent copies of the entire collection would cost only $1 million (1967 dollars) (48). In the long run the expense of converting to microfilm may be compensated for by the savings that would result from the markedly diminished need to maintain enormous storage facilities. Nevertheless, the initial outlay of funds may retard the widespread use of microfilm. The other major problem is that although the quality of table microfilm readers has improved in recent years, satisfactory portable models have yet to be devised. Presently, books and journals are definitely easier to carry around and read than is microfilm. In the future, however, a computer could rapidly locate the microfilm page, enlarge it to full size or scan it electronically, and transmit it over telephone wires, microwave, coaxial cables, or interactive television (48).

Another solution to the space dilemma is to utilize electronic storage techniques. These methods are preferable to microfilm because they provide more flexible information processing by using computers to locate text as well as to afford a base for programmed instruction. Access time to electronically stored information is less than that of microform, and therefore, faster searches can be conducted. Stored material can be quickly disseminated over national or local television networks. Whether microfilm or electronic storage techniques will be more economical may determine which method ultimately prevails (48).

The use of either of these methods does not mean that the HSIC of the future will be totally devoid of printed materials. However, instead of the current situation in which numerous volumes are accumulated, only the most frequently consulted books and periodicals would be stored in an HSIC. To purchase rarely utilized materials will be senseless, when they can be inexpensively, readily, and rapidly retrieved electronically from other facilities. If a reader wishes a permanent copy of an article, he can have it duplicated directly from a television screen (26, 49). Long-distance xerography or some other telefacsimile procedure also could be used for this purpose (48).

In addition to offering rapid access to journal articles, the HSIC of the future may provide other useful benefits. *Continuous bibliographic services* would afford health care professionals with an up-dated list of publications. The reader would register with the librarian the names of topics that are of interest to him. Every month the HSIC automatically would send him the titles and abstracts of articles pertaining to these subjects. These would be compiled by the National Library of Medicine and transmitted electronically to the local HSIC upon the librarian's request. Eventually, this information could be conveyed directly to the consumer so that users immediately could obtain up-to-date bibliographies (48). Some readers are unable to survey the entire medical literature because many articles are written in foreign languages. To overcome this difficulty, staff members of an HSIC could provide *translation services* (48). In the more distant future computers that automatically translate foreign languages could be employed routinely. Despite their current limitations, these programs already exist, and they are expected to become more refined and available in the future (50).

Another potentially useful activity of an HSIC would be to provide *editorial services*. Before submitting articles for publication, authors could give their manuscript to the HSIC where the references would be verified, the citations would be checked for uniformity, and the article would be reviewed to improve its clarity, grammar, and style. The HSIC also could provide films, videotapes, CAI, simulation programs, and other "learning packages." The HSIC would be a total educational laboratory offering the user a wide variety of services (48).

The HSIC will differ from the conventional library not only functionally, but also geographically. Whereas traditional library services are provided within a single building, the HSIC would not have to be bound by these physical restrictions. The availability of computer terminals, phonovision, and interactive television within hospitals, clinics, and offices would allow practitioners to obtain medical information where they work. A number of advantages could accrue from decentralizing information retrieval services. For example, every hospital floor could have a computer terminal and an IATV unit that could transmit information requested by the user. The computer terminal could provide CAI, CAS, and information retrieval, while the IATV could show slides, films, and articles. Because these educational resources would be so convenient, the provision of HSIC services within a hospital also could enhance patient care. Presently, if a doctor has a particular question or is uncertain about the treatment of a patient, he often has to go to a library for the answer. Because this task is so time consuming, he may forego seeking or checking on the answer to his question. With the immediate accessibility of

HSIC services within a hospital he could have his questions answered promptly and treat the patient more knowledgeably and with greater certainty. The HSIC will also provide medics with instantaneous answers to their patients' questions in the Post-Physician Era. An additional asset of HSICs is that they could well play a vital role in educating the general public about medical matters.

PUBLIC EDUCATION. The value of having a medically sophisticated public is self-evident. Ideally, everyone should know how to use clinical facilities appropriately, to eat and exercise properly, and to monitor their own health carefully. Forecasting that automation will play a major role in medicine's future, Ehrich Fromm worries:

> the individual will be so completely conditioned to submit to machines that he will lose the capacity to take care of his health in an active, responsible way. He will run to the "health service" whenever he has a physical problem, and he will lose the ability to observe his own physical processes, to discern changes, and to consider remedies for himself, even simple ones of keeping a diet or doing the right kind of exercise (51, pp. 110–111).

Conventional wisdom suggests that Fromm's dire prophecy can be averted by launching extensive and vigorous public education campaigns. Nevertheless, their effectiveness has not been substantiated.

Whenever our society detects a health problem, it unleashes a flurry of educational programs without seriously considering if these endeavors will alleviate or aggravate the problem. When illegal drug use reached epidemic proportions, popular magazines flooded the public with lurid photographs and stories in the hope of dissuading potential abusers. Regardless of how well-intended, these articles merely seemed to entice youth to take even more drugs. Schools embarked upon drug education classes, only to discover that they failed to modify the drug habits of their students (52). Public education efforts to foster more tolerant and constructive attitudes toward the mentally ill have also been disappointing. For example, two economically and culturally similar Canadian prairie towns with populations of approximately 1500 and 1100 were studied carefully to determine the effects of a massive public mental health information program. The larger town was inundated with literature, weekly radio programs, frequent Parent-Teacher Association discussion groups, a film festival, newspaper stories, and so on—all of which extolled the virtues of an "enlightened" approach to mental illness. After six months 56 percent of the people had been exposed to and were aware of the program's message. The smaller town, which was used as a control group, did not receive these programs. Questionnaires administered to members of both communities before and after the experimental period revealed that the public's attitude toward the mentally ill and psychiatric treatment were unaffected by the program (53). Another study conducted in the United States has also demonstrated that public mental health information has had a minimal impact upon popular attitudes (54). Not only have these educational activities had an insignificant effect, but some authorities suggest that they may even be harmful (55). Although this hypothesis has not been verified, an excessive focus upon public health education could generate a nation of psychosomatic cripples.

Of course, the potential value of public education projects should not be dismissed. The failure of most public health information programs may be the result of how they are performed and to whom they are directed. Psychiatrist Maxwell Jones is skeptical about the effectiveness of community-wide public relations campaigns that preach an "enlightened" approach to mental disease. He argues that educational programs can be useful if they are aimed at those who are affected rather than at a mass audience (56).

This view also could be debated. For example, according to the American Cancer Society, although cigarette sales have climbed to an all-time high of 585 billion in 1973, due to population growth, *per capita* cigarette consumption has declined by 32 percent since the Surgeon General issued his 1964 antismoking report. Whether this reduction was due to adverse cigarette publicity or to other factors remains unanswered. Before the Surgeon General's report, per capita cigarette consumption declined by 21 percent from 1953 to 1963. Thus, the post-report reduction of cigarette smoking may represent a mere acceleration of a previously existing trend, rather than a direct response to anticigarette publicity. Moreover, although since 1963 smokers over 17 years old have been decreasing, those under 17 have been increasing (57). In view of all this contradictory evidence, the effectiveness of public health education remains debatable. Certainly, the question deserves further study before we invest millions of dollars on the assumption that public education leads to public learning and that public learning leads to changing health-related behaviors. Although it is too early for a definitive verdict as to the value of public education, it is not too premature to consider methods by which this can be accomplished.

Information about how to maintain one's health (e.g., proper diet, adequate exercise) and ways to detect early signs of disease (e.g., periodic breast self-examination) should continue to be an important component of public educational endeavors. Whereas these topics have always been considered to be important, in the future other issues may deserve increasing attention. For example, the citizenry will need to be aware of how social and technological changes will alter health care delivery services (58–59). They will need to be familiar with the values and limitations of physician's assistants, computer-generated diagnoses and treatments, and multiphasic screening procedures. In view of the increasing complexity and changing character of the health care system, information about the appropriate use of clinical facilities will be especially important.

Biomedical innovations and their ethical implications will also deserve greater public attention. The rate at which these advances will be made could foster the belief that medical science can accomplish almost anything. The discrepancy between public expectations and clinical reality could lead to a disappointed, if not resentful, citizenry who will be reluctant to support medical services, education, and research. To avert this negative reaction, health care professionals should alert the public to what they can accomplish and what they *cannot* accomplish (60). Public education programs must differentiate between medical fact and moral conviction. When the Budapest city authorities established a public telephone answering service to disseminate sex information, they claimed that sex with anyone other than a marriage partner was "absolutely wrong" and that homosexuality was extremely dangerous (61). Although public health education programs should not necessarily exclude moral and ethical judgments, they should be identified as opinions instead of as facts.

In addition to the usual newspaper articles and television programs, technological advances may allow for the development of innovative vehicles for public health education. The San Bernardino County Medical Society has established a "Tel-Med" project by which people can telephone toll-free and request to hear a three- to eight-minute tape recording on a selected medical subject. Callers can choose from among 350 to 500 different tapes which cover a wide range of topics. They can obtain reliable information anonymously at no cost and without the need to ask embarrassing questions. For example, teenagers can ask for Tel-Med tapes on venereal disease, pregnancy, and drug abuse. The program has been extremely popular and is now being used throughout the country. The American Medical Association has provided $15,000 to translate the tapes into Spanish and to develop specific tapes for hospitalized patients (62).

In the more distant future information on selected topics could be obtained by interactive television (63). Eventually unidirectional (conventional) television will offer anywhere from 80 to 200 channels (64). One of these could be devoted exclusively to medical subjects by offering programs for both professionals and laymen. Already the Federal Communications Commission has licensed a private firm to produce and broadcast television shows for physicians in six major eastern cities (65). The content of these programs could be modified and expanded for a more general audience. With the increased use of communications satellites, unidirectional as well as bidirectional television programs dealing with a wide variety of medical subjects could eventually be relayed to any village on the globe (66).

HSICs, with their vast human and technological resources, would be especially well equipped to serve as centers for the health education of the general community. School children, church groups, and other interested parties could come to an HSIC where entertaining and informative programs could be presented on selected topics, just as planetariums presently offer the public lectures on astronomy. Unfortunately, many people may not be exposed to these programs if they have to go to the HSIC itself. If they will not come to the HSIC, the HSIC may have to come to them. Traveling "medical informationmobiles" could go into the community to present films and distribute literature. They also could use their television facilities to broadcast programs to local viewers.

Only future historians will be able to know when and if any of the developments mentioned in this chapter materialize. Meanwhile, because men are able to control their destinies to some extent, we must begin to select from a variety of options. The availability of so many choices represents a mixed blessing. It affords man the opportunity to construct his future from among many alternatives. However, he may become as immobilized as Buriden's ass who, while standing between two appetizing piles of hay, was unable to decide from which one to partake and eventually died of starvation (67). If we are not to become paralyzed by the abundance of options, we will have to make some critical decisions about tomorrow.

NOTES

1. Burwell, S. (1956). In G. W. Pickering "The Purpose of Medical Education." *British Medical Journal*, 2:113–116.
2. Culliton, B. J. (1974). "Medical Education: Institute Puts A Price on Doctors' Heads." *Science*, 185(4131):1272–1274.
3. Bradford, W. D. (1973). "Requirements for Admission to Medical School."

In J. Graves (ed.), *The Future of Medical Education*. Durham, N. C.: Duke University Press. Pp. 53–69.

4. Kahana, R. J., and G. L. Bibring (1964). "Personality Types in Medical Management." In N. E. Zinberg (ed.), *Psychiatry and Medical Practice in A General Hospital*. New York: International Universities Press. Pp. 108–123.

5. Zborowski, M. (1952). "Cultural Components in Responses to Pain." *Journal of Social Issues*, 8(4):16–30.

6. Mechanic, D. (1972). *Public Expectations and Health Care: Essays on the Changing Organization of Health Services*. New York: Wiley-Interscience.

7. Korsch, B. M., and V. F. Neguete (1972). "Doctor-Patient Communication." *Scientific American*, 227(2):66–74.

8. Field, M. G. (1971). "The Health Care System of Industrial Society: The Disappearance of the General Practitioner and Some Implications." In E. Mendelsohn, J. P. Swazey, and I. Taviss (eds.), *Human Aspects of Biomedical Innovation*. Cambridge; Harvard University Press. Pp. 156–180.

9. Balint, M. (1957). *The Doctor, His Patient, and the Illness*. New York: International Universities Press.

10. LeBow, M. D. (1973). *Behavior Modification: A Significant Method in Nursing Practice*. Englewood Cliffs, N. J.: Prentice-Hall.

11. Zinberg, N. E. (ed.) (1964). *Psychiatry and Medical Practice in A General Hospital*. New York: International Universities Press.

12. Suess, J. F. (1973). "Teaching Psychodiagnosis and Observation by Self-Instructional Programmed Videotapes." *Journal of Medical Education*, 48: 676–683.

13. Forrest, D. V., J. H. Ryan, R. Glavin, and H. H. Merritt (1974). "Through the Viewing Tube: Videocassette Psychiatry." *American Journal of Psychiatry*, 131:90–94.

14. Alger, I. (1973). "Audio-Visual Techniques in Family Therapy." In D. Bloch (ed.), *Techniques of Family Psychotherapy*. New York: Grune & Stratton. Pp. 65–73.

15. Stoeckle, J. D., A. Lazare, C. Weingarten, and M. T. McGuire (1971). "Learning Medicine by Videotaped Recordings." *Journal of Medical Education*, 46:518–524.

16. Birdwhistell, R. L. (1970). *Kinesics and Context: Essays on Body Motion Communication*. Philadelphia: University of Pennsylvania Press.

17. Scheflen, A. E. (1964). "The Significance of Posture in Communication Systems." *Psychiatry*, 27:316–331.

18. *Footnotes to the Future* (1974). "Forecasting the Future: The Future of Videotape," 4(6):1.

19. Dashef, S. S., W. M. Espey, and J. A. Lazarus (1974). "Time-Limited Sensitivity Groups for Medical Students." *American Journal of Psychiatry*, 131:287–292.

20. Strauss, M. B. (ed.) (1968). *Familiar Medical Quotations*. Boston: Little, Brown.

21. Halleck, S. L. (1974). "Legal and Ethical Aspects of Behavior Control." *American Journal of Psychiatry*, 131:381–385.

22. Maxmen, J. S., G. J. Tucker, and M. D. LeBow (1974). *Rational Hospital Psychiatry: The Reactive Environment*. New York: Brunner/Mazel.

23. Fordyce, W. E., R. S. Fowler, J. F. Lehmann, and B. J. DeLateur (1968). "Some Implications of Learning in Problems of Chronic Pain." *Journal of Chronic Diseases*, 21:179–190.

24. Skinner, B. F. (1972). *Beyond Freedom and Dignity*. Toronto: Bantam.

25. Levin, G., G. Hirsch, and E. Roberts (1971). "Narcotics and the Community: A Systems Simulation." *American Journal of Public Health*, 62: 861–873.

26. Kemeny, J. G. (1972). *Man and the Computer*. New York: Scribner's.

27. Thies, R., W. G. Harless, N. C. Lucas, and E. D. Jacobson (1969). "An Experiment Comparing Computer-Assisted Instruction with Lecture Presentation in Physiology." *Journal of Medical Education*, 44:1156–1160.

28. Friedman, R. B. (1973). "A Computer Program for Simulating the Patient-Physician Encounter." *Journal of Medical Education*, 48:92–97.

29. Penta, F. B., and S. Kofman (1973). "The Effectiveness of Simulation Devices in Teaching Selected Skills of Physical Diagnosis." *Journal of Medical Education*, 48:442–445.

30. Hoffer, E. P., G. O. Barnett, and B. B. Farquhar (1972). "Computer Simulation Model for Teaching Cardio-Pulmonary Resuscitation." *Journal of Medical Education*, 47:343–348.

31. Harless, W. G., G. G. Drennon, J. J. Marxer, J. A. Root, and G. E. Miller (1971). "CASE: A Computer-Aided Simulation of the Clinical Encounter." *Journal of Medical Education*, 46:443–448.

32. Goldberg, M., S. B. Green, M. L. Moss, C. B. Marbach, and D. Garfinkel (1973). "Computer-Based Instruction and Diagnosis of Acid-Base Disorders." *Journal of the American Medical Association*, 223:269–275.

33. Harless, W. G., G. G. Drennon, J. J. Marxer, J. A. Root, L. L. Wilson, and G. E. Miller (1973). "CASE—A Natural Language Computer Model." *Computers in Biology and Medicine*, 3:227–246.

34. Brigham, C. R., and M. Kamp (1974). "The Current Status of Computer-Assisted Instruction in the Health Sciences." *Journal of Medical Education*, 49:278–279.

35. London, I. M. (1973). "The College and University in Medical Education." In J. Graves (ed.), *The Future of Medical Education*. Durham, N. C.: Duke University Press. Pp. 43–51.

36. Van Der Kloot, W. G. (1973). "The Education of Biomedical Scientists." In J. Graves (ed.), *The Future of Medical Education*. Durham, N. C.: Duke University Press. Pp. 87–105.

37. Flexner, A. (1910). *Medical Education in the United States and Canada*. A Report to the Carnegie Foundation for the Advancement of Teaching. Bulletin 4. Boston: Updyke.

38. Brown, R. E. (1973). "Financing Medical Education." In J. Graves (ed.), *The Future of Medical Education*. Durham, N. C.: Duke University Press. Pp. 173–192.

39. McLaughlin, C. P., and A. Sheldon (1974). *The Future and Medical Care: A Health Manager's Guide to Forecasting*. Cambridge, Mass.: Ballinger.

40. Handler, P. (ed.) (1970). *Biology and the Future of Man*. New York: Oxford University Press.

41. Meadows, D. H., D. L. Meadows, J. Randers, and W. W. Behrens III (1972). *The Limits to Growth: A Report for the Club of Rome's Project on the Predicament of Mankind*. New York: Universe.

42. Brown, H. (1954). *The Challenge of Man's Future*. New York: Viking.

43. Licklider, J. C. R. (1965). *Libraries of the Future*. Cambridge: M.I.T. Press.

44. Cummings, M. M. (1973). "Publications: Progress or Pollution." *American Scientist*, 61:163–166.

45. Fiore, Q. (1972). "The Future of the Book." In H. Yaker, H. Osmond, and F. Cheek (eds.), *The Future of Time: Man's Temporal Environment*. Garden City, N. J.: Doubleday. Pp. 479–497.

46. McCarn, D. B. (1973). "Data Bases and the National Library of Medicine." Paper delivered at the New England Regional Group of the Medical Library Association, Hanover, N. H. September 14.

47. *Yale Medicine* (1972). "MEDLINE at the Yale Medical Library," 7(3):16.

48. Miller, J. G. (1967). "Design for A University Health Sciences Information Center." *Journal of Medical Education*, 42:404–429.

49. Hellman, H. (1969). *Communications in the World of the Future*. New York: Evans.

50. Fink, D. G. (1966). *Computers and the Human Mind*. Garden City, N. J.: Doubleday.

51. Fromm, E. (1968). *The Revolution of Hope: Toward A Humanized Technology*. Toronto: Bantam.

52. Weaver, S. C., and F. S. Tennant (1973). "Effectiveness of Drug Education Programs for Secondary School Students." *American Journal of Psychiatry*, 130:812–814.

53. Cumming, E., and J. Cumming (1957). *Closed Ranks: An Experiment in Mental Health Education*. Cambridge: Harvard University Press.

54. Star, S. A. (1957). "The Place of Psychiatry in Popular Thinking." Paper delivered to the meeting of the American Association for Public Opinion Research, Washington, D. C. May 9.

55. Werkö, L. *Health—Present Concepts and Future*. Mimeo.

56. Jones, M. (1968). *Social Psychiatry in Practice: The Idea of the Therapeutic Community*. Baltimore: Penguin.

57. *The Futurist* (1974). "Smoking: Per Capita Cigarette Consumption Declines in U. S." 8:210.

58. Schwartz, W. B. (1970). "Medicine and the Computer: The Promise and Problems of Change." *New England Journal of Medicine*, 283:1257–1264.

59. Perry, J. W. (1969). "Career Mobility in Allied Health Education." *Journal of the American Medical Association*, 210:107–110.

60. Cherkasky, M. (1973). "Medical Education and Practice—Circa 1985." In J. Graves (ed.), *The Future of Medical Education*. Durham, N. C.: Duke University Press. Pp. 3–26.

61. *Medical Tribune and Medical News* (1972). " Hello: I've Got A Sexy Query'; Budapest Telephone Answers," 13(48):1.

62. *American Medical News* (1973). " 'Tel-Med' Puts Health Advice As Close As the Telephone," 16(13):14.

63. *The Futurist* (1972). "Information Technology and its Implications," 6:244–249.

64. Bagdikian, B. H. (1971). "How Much More Communication Can We Stand?" *The Futurist*, 5:180–183.

65. *Medical World News* (1972). "National TV 'Narrowcast' for MDs," 13(45): 4–5.

66. Brown, L. R. (1972). "New Supranational Institutions." *The Futurist*, 6: 197–202.

67. Lipowski, Z. J. (1970). "The Conflict of Buridan's Ass or Some Dilemmas of Affluence: The Theory of Attractive Stimulus Overload." *American Journal of Psychiatry*, 127:273–279.

8

TOWARDS
A NEW IDENTITY_____

Although this book is primarily about future interrelationships
between man, medicine, and technology, its speculations
may have more extensive implications. Because neither man,
medicine, nor technology exists in a vacuum, one cannot explore
the future of the American health care system without touching
upon more global psychological, social, and historical issues.
Similarly, this book has not been written in isolation; it and its
author have been exposed to the social and psychohistorical forces
that have emerged during its preparation over the past five years.
Although I made every effort not to be *unduly* swayed by present-
day events and attitudes, undoubtedly they have tainted my projections. In this chapter I discuss briefly how current psychological,
social, and historical developments may influence some more
global aspects of the future that are suggested by the emergence
of a Post-Physician Era.

To maintain the generally optimistic tone of this book may be
incongruous, considering the events of the last five years. During
this time we have become progressively disillusioned by our

apparent incapacity to resolve an unrelenting succession of man-
made dilemmas—from Vietnam, to alienated youth, to drug
abuse, to racism, to ecology, to an energy shortage, to Watergate,
to inflation, and to a recession. We scurry from crisis to crisis, not
because we have mastered the preceding one, but only because
the next one suddenly appears more ominous. Our despair at
failing to overcome these problems becomes compounded as we
sense that the solutions we attempt to employ are either hopelessly
inadequate or create more difficulties than they resolve. The
faith we allegedly once possessed in the ability of our politicians,
intellectuals, and institutions to contend with the quandaries of
modern society is declining rapidly. Given the pessimism of the
present, the hopeful view of the future presented in this book may
appear as a last hurrah of a sinking civilization.

An undercurrent of futility also exists in regard to the problems
of contemporary American medicine. For years we have been
inundated with exposés about the maldistribution and shortage
of doctors, the ineffectiveness of our health care system vis-à-vis
the other industrialized nations, and the spiraling costs of clinical
care which pays for thousands of unnecessary hospital beds,
specialized treatment units, operations, and medications. There
are no lack of villains in these exposés—the American Medical
Association, the American Hospital Association, the pharmaceutical companies, the insurance industry, avaricious physicians,
greedy malpractice attornies, opportunistic politicians, soft-headed
humanists, and cold-blooded technocrats. There also is an abundance of ideological explanations for our current dilemmas—
specialization, "progress," science, racism, sexism, capitalism, and
socialism. Our choice of villains often determines our choice of
solutions. Depending upon who or what is blamed, the alleged
salvation of our health care system rests either with socializing
medicine, federalizing health insurance, altering the malpractice
system, restoring free enterprise, nationalizing the pharmaceutical industry, rejuvenating the family doctor, establishing community control, and on and on. Why then, with so many
allegedly available proposals do we still feel impotent to handle
the American health care crisis?

Admittedly, the answers to this question rest partially with the facts that the issues are complex, no single solution is sufficient, and there is no consensus on the optimal approach. Criteria for what constitutes adequate health care are not precise and universally accepted, and the standards that do exist are continually escalating. If medicine were practiced today as it was a hundred years ago, it would now be labeled as unacceptable. Nevertheless, I suspect that a significant aspect of the difficulty in designing an effective health care system for the future has been our failure to examine a fundamental assumption: The doctor is essential for the delivery of medical services. Despite the innumerable scholarly critiques on the health care system, all of them have accepted the myth of physician necessity. Although they have challenged the doctor's technical, monetary, organizational, and ethical practices, they have never questioned the need for his existence. Consequently, this lack of imagination has restricted the range of future options that have been considered. Given the severity of our health care problems, why do we cling to the belief that the doctor is a necessity? Why has a medic-computer model never been proposed despite its potentially enormous value?

In prescientific societies priests, barber-surgeons, apothecaries, and next door neighbors frequently provided health care services. During the last few centuries physicians and at times other highly trained professionals have been deemed the only ones sufficiently knowledgeable to preserve health and prolong life. Our survival has become psychologically and inextricably linked to the survival of the doctor. Because advocating a return to prescientific medical practice would be absurd, every proposal aimed at resolving our health care dilemmas presupposes that physicians must be an integral and necessary component of the plan. This belief was justified as long as doctors and other allied health personnel were the only ones capable of making diagnostic and treatment decisions. Now the technological revolution affords us with a genuine alternative to this line of reasoning.

The general unwillingness to recognize the full impact that computers will play upon the delivery of health care reveals a great deal not only about medicine, but also about contemporary society. It highlights what I suspect future historians will view as one of the most vital issues of the 20th century—the profound need to redefine man's limitations and unique abilities.

Throughout history the question of what constitutes man's special qualities has been one of his major preoccupations. For centuries the issue took the form of inquiring how he differed from other animals. This subject was philosophically important because it helped clarify the nature of man and define his uniqueness. The exploration of this issue also had psychological benefits because, in describing how man differed from other species, man could point to qualities, such as the capacity for language and abstract thought, that helped to elevate his self-esteem by emphasizing his superiority. Although today the question of man's distinctions from animals does not generate a great deal of passion, humanity's concern with his own superiority has been resurrected by the advent of the technological revolution.

As unsettling as it may be, computers can perform a wide range of activities more efficiently and effectively than man. They can rapidly calculate enormously complicated mathematical equations, store and retrieve vast quantities of information, and similate complex human and social systems. That computers are able to conduct these operations is generally recognized; that machines can execute many "creative" tasks is less widely known. Computers have been programmed to compose music with both 16th century counterpoint and modern 12-tone styles and also to incorporate a variety of rhythms and dynamics. Although with less sophistication, machines can translate languages and write poetry. When 100 people were asked to compare reproductions of a genuine Mondrian painting with a Mondrian-like picture generated by a computer, 72 believed the real Mondrian was produced by the machine, and 59 aesthetically preferred the picture created by the computer (1). Previously I noted that a checker playing machine was even able to defeat its inventor (2–3). Of greater importance is that technological progress need not wait for man's next scientific breakthrough. *By themselves* computers are generating whole new families of machines for processing information, translating languages, communicating data, and so on. In the future they may be able to pursue objectives which man himself does not realize exist (4). I mention these points not with the intent of proposing that the computer is always superior to man, * but only to suggest that it is able to perform an impressive array of activities that formerly only man himself felt capable of conducting. Computers have replaced animals as the yardstick against which man attempts to measure and thereby proclaim his superiority. The enormous capabilities and impact of the computer threatens man's belief in his own omnipotence. Every day we hear about men being replaced by machines. Recently I saw a bittersweet cartoon of a woman explaining that her scientist-husband became dejected upon discovering that he had just lost the Nobel Prize to a computer.

Because machines will be able to outperform doctors in the execution of diagnostic and treatment tasks, the prospect of a Post-Physician Era also challenges man's assumed superiority. Despite its many advantages, the introduction of medical computers will generate resentment because, among other reasons, it will confront man with the realization that he is not so unique, special, superior, or necessary as he would like to believe. Of course, the computer is not the first scientific discovery that has threatened man's pride. Science has forced him to acknowledge that his earth is not the center of the universe and that his creation was not God's first order of business. Indeed, the history of science has continually undermined man's faith in his own superiority and confronted him with his own limitations. Despite all the omnipotence we ascribe to doctors, the real possibility of a Post-Physician Era painfully reminds us of these facts.

Just as medical computers underscore the limits of physicians, so too will future biomedical innovations highlight humanity's biological deficiencies. The anticipated ability to manipulate genetic material, create an artificial placenta, and clone superior beings illustrates that technology could improve upon man's reproductive processes. In the future synthetic organs will be

---

* Authoritative discussions comparing men and computers can be found elsewhere (1, 4–7).

able to outperform natural ones. Eventually, human-machine chimeras may be able to exceed man's physical powers, emotional functions, and intellectual capacities. These innovations may seem frightening because of their potential dehumanizing effect and impact upon man's evolutionary future. Condemning these innovations, however, can neither sweep away the fact of their possible development nor allow us to avoid recognizing the biological limitations of our species.

There also is little point in saying that there is really nothing new in modern technology because the use of technology is almost as old as man himself. To do so would be like dismissing the impact of Freud, just because Sophocles and Shakespeare demonstrated an awareness of unconscious motivations. Although early Christian communal theorists and pre-Marxian historians considered economic factors, these facts do not vitiate the force of Marx's economic determinism (4). What is new and important about modern technology is that it permeates and changes almost every aspect of contemporary experience. Because we can neither flee from its social and personal impact nor ignore its enormous potential, it obstinately confronts man with his own limitations.

If the future of medicine and technology will force man to acknowledge new areas in which he is deficient, how then can he learn to live with this discomforting realization? Although I do not have any satisfactory answers to this question, several thoughts may deserve consideration.

The recognition of man's limitations need not detract from his dignity. It could serve as a stimulus for him to redefine the nature of that dignity. To believe we can surpass the machine where in reality we cannot will be destructive to the human spirit. If, under the guise of humanism, we continue to force man to conduct tasks that computers can do better, we will be making machines of ourselves. A heightened awareness of our limitations vis-à-vis the computer provides us with a fresh opportunity to examine realistically both our relative deficiencies and, more importantly, our relative advantages over the machine. A medic-computer model has been proposed partially with this notion in mind. With the advent of this development, those tasks best performed by machines will be done by machines; those best performed by humans will be done by humans. Undoubtedly, as science evolves, this relative distribution of labor will change. But as it changes, we will have to recognize and distinguish continually the areas in which technology is superior from the areas in which man is superior.

Another lesson underscored by the prospect of a Post-Physician Era is the growing symbiotic nature of man and machine (8). Man is neither fully dependent on the machine, nor is the machine fully dependent on man. Instead, an interdependent relationship exists between them. Each needs the other. This relationship need not be a competitive one. If man needs to compete, let him compete with himself. Let him improve upon his past by fulfilling his potential. Let him maximize his *unique characteristics*, such as the capacity for *wisdom*, *morality*, and *nobility*, and let him utilize technology to capitalize upon these qualities.

Many will argue that the expanded use of automation will render man so dependent upon technology that he will be forced to compromise his wisdom, morality, and nobility to adjust to the demands of a computerized society. Many claim that this has already occurred (9–10). Even the most avid technophil would have to admit to a kernel of truth in these assertions. Whether one speaks of an automated society in general or a Post-Physician Era in particular, the development of both these events will introduce a certain degree of conformity and inflexibility. For example, once the doctor becomes obsolete, reverting to a physician-centered model will be nearly impossible, even if some individuals would strongly prefer it. However, to believe that an automated society is the only one that breeds conformity and denies flexibility would be a mistake. Throughout history man has been subject to the tyrannical dictates of his environment. Whereas in primitive times he had to adjust to the whims of nature, today he has to conform to the norms, values, and institutions of contemporary civilization. All societies—past, present, and future—demand human compromise. The only differences between historical eras are the kinds of compromises that are required of man in order to survive. Moreover, his need to compromise does not preclude his taking advantage of the opportunities to practice his morality, nobility, and wisdom. Regardless of societal constraints, he is still free to choose from among numerous options in conducting his life. The nature of his choices will determine the quality of his existence. Unfortunately, in an attempt to rationalize his failures, contemporary man often ignores the realistic opportunities before him and claims he is being dehumanized and victimized by technology. Scapegoating automation is a copout; it will bring neither solutions to the problems of the world nor salvation to the problems of the spirit. The chance to accomplish these objectives could materialize if we learn to live in harmony with the new technology. If we are able to recognize and accept the realistic limits and the unique abilities of both man and machine, we may be able to face the future with greater optimism than we do at present.

Whether this hope will materialize depends partially upon man's willingness to exercise his wisdom, morality, and nobility in shaping the future. This future is neither fixed nor preordained; today's policies will inevitably form tomorrow's realities. In large measure the future of our choice is within our power. Of course, there is no consensus as to what our future should be like; one man's utopia may be another's dystopia. If one shares my belief that a Post-Physician Era and the other proposals advanced in this book are worthy of accomplishment, then we should begin planning to implement them *now*. I stress the word *now* not because catastrophies will result if we fail to act today, but rather because the longer we delay the harder it will be to overcome the inertia and despair currently prevailing within our society.

If the predictions I have suggested materialize, 50 years from now many individuals may view the current methods of the physician as hopelessly antiquated. For example, they might say that to believe that by thumping on a chest one could accurately evaluate the size of the heart is a primitive notion more likely possessed by a medicine man than by a man of medicine. Nevertheless, future historians may fondly look back upon the doctor. They may record that despite his archaic techniques, he frequently was a sympathetic, creative, intelligent, and at times even an ingenious practitioner. They may recognize that without his willingness to train paraprofessionals and to develop automated clinical programs, a medic-computer model would never have emerged. His greatest legacy may be that he made these contributions to the more humane health care delivery system that will exist under the New Medical Order of the 21st century.

NOTES

1. Apter, M. J. (1970). *The Computer Simulation of Behaviour*. New York: Harper Colophon Books.

2. Samuel, A. L. (1959). "Some Studies in Machine Learning Using the Game of Checkers." *IBM Journal of Research and Development*, 3:210–229.

3. Samuel, A. L. (1967). "Some Studies in Machine Learning Using the Game of Checkers. II—Recent Progress." *IBM Journal of Research and Development*, 11:601–617.

4. Diebold, J. (1970). *Man & the Computer: Technology As an Agent of Social Change*. New York: Avon.

5. Fink, D. G. (1966). *Computers and the Human Mind*. Garden City, N. J.: Doubleday.

6. Toffler, A. (1971). *Future Shock*. New York: Bantam.

7. Muller, H. J. (1970). *The Children of Frankenstein: A Primer on Modern Technology and Human Values*. Bloomington: Indiana University Press.

8. Kemeny, J. G. (1972). *Man and the Computer*. New York: Scribner's.

9. Ellul, J. (1964). *The Technological Society*. New York: Vintage.

10. Roszak, T. (1968). *The Making of the Counter Culture: Reflections on the Technocratic Society and Its Youthful Opposition*. Garden City, N. J.: Doubleday.

APPENDIX A

CRITICAL ELEMENTS
IN FUTURES RESEARCH⸻

Futures research involves more than simply choosing objectives and finding techniques to achieve them. Any postulated alternative future must have a chance of occurring. For example, although one *could* predict that by 1980 nurses will routinely perform open heart surgery, this estimate would be of little value. There is no evidence that by 1980 nurses will have developed the necessary skills nor that surgeons will relinquish their authority to perform these operations. Thus, the existence of data to support the possible occurrence of a projected future will enhance the possibility of it materializing. Although predictions without evidence to support them may be thought provoking, they belong more in the realm of fantasy than in the province of serious and scholarly futures research.

An optimal forecast must reflect an awareness of at least nine critical elements: intrafield relatedness, interfield relatedness, immediate versus enduring trends, specificity, economic parameters, psychological factors, consequences, value explicitness, and clearly articulated assumptions (1). Although thoroughly

266

considering these nine factors in performing futures research does not guarantee an accurate forecast, their use will enhance the value of a projection. Furthermore, the reader can utilize these criteria in evaluating the quality of a prediction (1–3).

INTRAFIELD RELATEDNESS. Developments in one sector of a field may affect trends in another area within the same general field. For example, the diminishing number of general practitioners has contributed to the increased utilization of hospital emergency rooms (4). This criterion suggests that a forecasted event will not remain static if a development that affects it is evolving.

INTERFIELD RELATEDNESS. A projection should include consideration of events in areas that, although not usually associated with the item under examination, nevertheless could affect it. A group of Maine physicians were asked which development of the past 50 years most contributed to improved health care. Some doctors suggested the laboratory synthesis of insulin, while others proposed the use of cortisone. One physician, however, felt the availability of improved highways, which provided patients with greater access to doctors and hospitals, was the most significant development (5). Thus, in projecting alternative medical futures one needs to identify the effects that trends occurring outside of medicine may have upon developments happening within medicine.

IMMEDIATE VERSUS ENDURING TRENDS. A forecast should not be influenced excessively by recent developments which may not necessarily persist or, even if they do, not have any lasting significance. For example, having noted the liberated sexual attitudes of many contemporary youth, Leo Davids has predicted that by 1990, polygamous, polyandrous, and group marriages will become commonplace (6). Without other collaborative evidence, however, I would suggest that this projection overestimates the importance of a current fad by automatically assuming it will become an enduring social pattern. An optimal forecast must distinguish what is relevant from what is topical (1).

SPECIFICITY. A forecast is only as good as the details it contains. It is necessary to indicate specifically the exact nature of an anticipated development, as well as the precise date it is expected to occur. Such specificity is useful to prepare adequately to cope with the consequences of a future event and to correlate it with the occurrence of other future developments.

ECONOMIC PARAMETERS. The costs of any social, technological, or medical innovation must be considered to project future developments. This factor is especially important in the field of health care, where fiscal realities rather than medical needs often determine the availability of treatment. For example, in 1971 renal dialysis, a life-sustaining procedure for patients in kidney failure, frequently cost over $44,000 per year. Until more economical means of treating these individuals are discovered, it would be unlikely that a sufficient number of renal dialysis units will be established to save the lives of the 7000 to 8000 patients who annually die from kidney disorders (7). At times unexpected consequences can result from economic policies. For instance, large numbers of elderly couples have been living together because social security payments are reduced when two people get married (8). The point is that monetary factors significantly influence if and when a particular event or trend will emerge.

PSYCHOLOGICAL FACTORS. The degree to which people will promote or deter the emergence of a particular development depends partially upon a myriad of psychological forces. Although attitudinal and behavioral variables must be considered in futures research, psychological "evidence" must be carefully scrutinized. Psychological factors often are difficult to identify, hard to prove, open to a wide variety of interpretations, and are fluctuating constantly in a rapidly evolving society. One must be leery of assuming that commonly held or avant-garde beliefs about psychological issues are valid. For example, psychology professor Lawrence Casler writes, "Marriage, for *most* people, has outlived its usefulness and is doing more harm than good" (italics added) (9). Although this view is held by many people and may even contain a grain of truth, it is not substantiated by more objective data. Instead, there is solid evidence that nonmarried individuals have a higher rate of schizophrenia, depression, and suicide (10). Although I do not mean to underestimate the importance of emotional and subjective factors in futures research, the reader must distinguish between psychological speculation and psychological fact.

CONSEQUENCES. An optimal forecast specifies and evaluates thoroughly all of the potential consequences of a projected event. Not only will the occurrence of a single development lead to the emergence of other events, but these events in turn may give rise to further developments. The following illustration is not offered as an argument against self-instructional aids, and its conclusions are not substantiated. It is provided *only* for the purpose of demonstrating how a single innovation may have far-flung and often unexpected consequences. If a medical school faculty primarily used self-instructional teaching machines to train its students, fewer lectures and small group discussions would occur (first order consequence). As a result, contact between students would be minimized (second order consequence), thereby reducing the opportunities for camaraderies to develop (third order consequence). This fraternization helps students to cope emotionally with the rigors of medical school; without it some of them may develop feelings of isolation, insecurity, anxiety, and depression (fourth-order consequence). In turn some students may drop out of school, and others may obtain psychiatric treatment

(fifth order consequences). What began as an educational innovation (i.e., the increased use of self-instructional aids) may lead
to consequences (i.e., increased dropout rate, increased use of
psychiatric services) that not only are far removed from the
initial development, but also were unlikely to have been considered originally (1).

VALUE EXPLICITNESS.   In projecting alternative futures the
investigator should evaluate and clearly state the relative desirability of any anticipated development. Innovations do not exist
in a value-free vacuum. Not all that is new is good, nor is all that
is old, bad. Moreover, every prediction is influenced by the values
of the person who formulated it (2). All too often, however, the
forecaster is not explicit in stating his own biases. Therefore, for
the reader to assess fully the conclusions of the investigator, the
former must be cognizant of the values of the latter.

CLEARLY ARTICULATED ASSUMPTIONS.   A   forecast
should list the assumptions upon which it is based. For example,
a prediction that medical schools will have to double their number
of graduates by 1990 to maintain current levels of health care is
based on the assumptions that a nuclear or ecological holocaust
will not occur in the interim. Furthermore, this forecast would be
predicated on the suppositions that the population will double, the
citizens will desire the same level of medical services, and computers and paraprofessionals will not perform a large proportion
of health care activities presently conducted by doctors. Because
a projection is only as good as the assumptions that went into
formulating it, a failure to state them explicitly may lead to
incorrect predictions and wasted planning.
    In evaluating the qualities of any prediction one should consider
all of these criteria systematically. Although forecasts that receive
high marks according to these factors are not necessarily accurate,
they are more likely to be accurate.

NOTES

1. Maxmen, J. S. (1975). "Forecasting and Medical Education." *Journal of Medical Education*, 50:54–65.

2. Amara, R. C., and G. R. Salancik (1972). "Forecasting: From Conjectural Art Toward Science." *The Futurist*, 6:112–117.

3. Bundy, R. F. "The Quality of Forecasts: Fakery or Freedom." Mimeo.

4. *Medical World News* (1970–1971). "Emergency Departments and the Non-Emergency Deluge," 11(62):23–28.

5. Sidel, V. W. (1971). "New Technologies and the Practice of Medicine." In E. Mendelsohn, J. P. Swazey, and I. Taviss (eds.), *Human Aspects of Biomedical Innovation*. Cambridge: Harvard University Press. Pp. 131–155.

6. Davids, L. (1971). "North American Marriage: 1990." *The Futurist*, 5: 190–194.

7. Greenberg, S. (1971). *The Quality of Mercy: A Report on the Critical Condition of Hospital and Medical Care in America*. New York: Atheneum.

8. Coates, J. F. (1971). "Technological Assessment: The Benefits . . . the Costs . . . the Consequences." *The Futurist*, 5:225–231.

9. Casler, L. (1975). "Permissive Matrimony: Proposals for the Future." *Reflections*, 10(1):15–30.

10. Detre, T., and H. Jarecki (1971). *Modern Psychiatric Treatment*. Philadelphia: Lippincott.

APPENDIX B
A CHRONOLOGY OF
THE FUTURE _____

As mentioned in Appendix A, one characteristic of a worthwhile forecast is *time specificity*. Table 3 indicates the dates by which I predict certain events will occur with a 50 percent probability. Details about these developments can be found in the body of the text. Some of the estimates in this table have been derived and occassionally modified from other sources (1–3), including a number of Delphi exercises (4–7), which are reiterated anonymous debates between experts (8). Nevertheless, I assume full responsibility for all of these forecasts. The meaning of the abbreviations used in the table are as follows:

AMA	American Medical Association
ANA	American Nurses' Association
CAI	Computer-aided instruction
CAS	Computer-aided simulation
CATV	Cable television
CCTV	Closed circuit television
CHS	College of health sciences
CNS	Central nervous system
COMSAT	Communications satellite

DNA	Desoxyribonucleic acid
EKG	Electrocardiogram
HSIC	Health science information center
H-TM*	Health-team model
IATV	Interactive television
IQ	Intelligence quotient
M-CM*	Medic-computer model
MD	Medical doctor
NHI	National health insurance
NLM	National Library of Medicine
NMDB	National medical data bank
PA	Physician's assistant
P-CM*	Physician-centered model
PSRO	Professional standards review organization
SMI	School of medical investigation
SMM	School of medical management
TV	Television
US	United States

* The percentages following these abbreviations in the table refer to the proportion of total health care services delivered by these models within the United States.

TABLE 5—PROJECTED DEVELOPMENTS RELATED TO MEDICINE

Year	Communication and Computer Technology	Biomedicine and Therapeutics	Education and Occupations	Miscellaneous
By 1980	Invention of wall-size TV	Development of useful tissue adhesives to replace sutures	"Rotating" and "straight" internships replaced by "flexible" and "categorical" internships	Wide use of generic substitution for brand name drugs
	Establishment of TV network for MDs			
	Extensive use of automated EKG interpretations	General availability of male contraceptive and long-acting female contraceptive drugs	Pharmacist's education stressing his consultant role	Laboratory creation of protein for food by in vitro cellular processes
	Use of computer-patient IQ testing			
	Introduction of IATV via COMSAT	Development of tests for rapid diagnosis of viral diseases	Unrestricted medical license granted only after completion of residency	Enactment of NHI covering 75 percent of medical costs
	Wide use of computers for hospital record storage and data retrieval	General availability of home diagnostic kits for urine and fecal examinations	Medical ethics a standard medical school course	Widely established PSROs
	Regional medical data computer banks established	Early determination of fetal sex with 90 percent accuracy	Average 45-hour work week for MDs	AMA membership below 40 percent of US MDs
	50 percent of US homes with CATV	Discovery of etiology of most leukemias	Ombudsmen widely used in hospitals and clinics	Annual per capita health costs in US: $670
	Routine use of CATV for medical conferences		MEDLINE-generated abstracts	Noncarcinogenic cigarette
			CAS and CAI in 80 percent of medical schools	

By 1985					
Long-hand computer input	Immunizing agents that protect against most viral agents available	Recertification required by 50 percent of specialty boards	Virtual cessation of diploma nursing schools	"No-fault" malpractice insurance	Decriminalization of marijuana
Wide use of computers for drug information services	Development of economically useful mass-administered contraceptive agents	Use of teaching machines that respond to a student's answers and to his physiologic state (tension)	5 percent of US MDs in a labor union	Legislation to ensure privacy of computer-stored data	Red Cross a semi-public agency in most nations
20 channels widely available with CATV	Artificial heart implantation	Virtual obsolescence of the general practitioner		P-CM = 80 percent	Annual per capita health costs in US: $850
Wide use of computers for requesting and evaluating lab tests	Chemical synthesis of specific antibodies	Wide use of IATV for clinical teaching conferences		H-TM = 20 percent	Government-established standards for medical computers
Wide use of videophones in hospitals	Laboratory solution of immunologic rejection problem	Computer and communication experts members of 90 percent of medical school faculties		M-CM = 0 percent	3.6 billion prescriptions filled in US
Intercity conference videophones for medical use	Development of reliable chemical tests for psychotic disorders				90 percent of medical costs covered by NHI
Establishment of nation-					

TABLE 3 (*Continued*)

Year	Communication and Computer Technology	Biomedicine and Therapeutics	Education and Occupations	Miscellaneous
	al computerized organ bank for transplants	Effective anticold vaccine	HSIC access from hospitals via IATV	P-CM = 55 percent
	CAI in home via IATV	Chemical treatment of gallstones	Some kind of continuing education for MD relicensure required by 50 percent of states	H-TM = 45 percent
	NMDB established	Drugs to raise IQ of borderline retardates by 10 to 20 points	The "classical" lecture system ended in 40 percent of medical schools by teaching machines, CCTV, IATV, and audio-visual aids	M-CM = 0 percent
	Wide use of computers for medical history taking	Wide application of drugs directly to diseased organs rather than orally	State licensure for psychotherapists regardless of discipline	
	First use of lasers for communication transmission	Wide use of implanted chemical capsules for preventing contraception	5 percent of MDs in solo practice	
	3-D TV available for commercial use	Capacity to detect many diseases in embryo	Editorial services in HSIC	
	Establishment of national medical TV network		Establishment of SMIs	
	Oral computer input		Wide use of PAs to deliver primary care and some specialized care	
	Portable telephone widely available			

276

By 1990			
Medico-legal information available via IATV	Development of artificial colon	Wide use of professional nurses to deliver primary care	Failure to consult a computer considered grounds for malpractice suit
Wide use of computers for monitoring devices attached directly to patients in their homes	Development of effective broad spectrum antiviral agents	40 percent of MD's time spent in direct patient care	Dismantlement of PSROs
Telephone network fully digitalized	Development of safe chemical means to reverse effects of arteriosclerosis	NLM able to transmit text to local HSICs	Water and air pollution problems largely diminished
Frequent use of "tele-medicine"	Chemical cure for schizophrenias	Single federal licensing system for MDs	Establishment of public computer utility
Wide use of computers to prescribe medications	Development of anti-cancer vaccines	50 percent of technical nurses have withdrawn from ANA and their own organization formed	Chemical synthesis of cheap nutritious food
Wide use of phonovision	Wide use of tests in children that will reliably predict their developing some major mental illnesses in adulthood	Establishment of SMMs	PAs have associate memberships in AMA
Medical records of 80 percent of US population stored in NMDB		HSIC access from home via IATV	Pharmaceutical industry nationalized
Wide use of general purpose computers in the home		Routine HSIC use of automated language translaters capable of coping with idiomatic complexities	P-CM = 25 percent
90 percent of urban homes with IATV		50 percent of PAs in labor union	H-TM = 75 percent
Some people able to have daily checkups of body			M-CM = 0 percent

TABLE 3 (*Continued*)

Year	Communication and Computer Technology	Biomedicine and Therapeutics	Education and Occupations	Miscellaneous
	functions by computer with preliminary analysis and warnings of impending illness		75 percent of the tasks of the traditional pharmacist performed by pharmacy technicians	
	All body fluids and functions routinely analyzed and diagnostic reports and summaries prepared by machines		Wide use of professional nurses and PAs to coordinate multiphasic screening procedures	
			Technical nurses play a major role in their own training programs	
			Literature directly obtainable from NLM via IATV	
By 1995	Invention of "pharmaceutical automat"	Development of drugs that alter memory and learning	85 percent of pharmacists working in hospitals and clinics rather than in drugstores	6000 hospitals in US
	CATV with 80 channels widely available	*In vitro* fertilization of human ovum with implantation into host mothers	Multidisciplinary planning for medic education	Techniques that permit useful exploitation of ocean through aquaculture farming, with the effect of producing 20 percent
	General availability of computers to conduct psychotherapy		25 percent of MD's time	

3-D TV widely used for home entertainment	Development of synthetic blood substitute	spent in direct patient care	of the world's caloric intake
Frequent use of conference videophones for group psychotherapy	General availability of physical and chemical means to modify some forms of criminal behavior	20 percent of US MDs in a labor union	P-CM = 10 percent
First experimental use of computers for all diagnostic and treatment decisions in patient care	First human clone		H-TM = 88 percent
Extensive use of IATV to monitor aged within their homes	Application of compulsory birth control in some nations without being effective		M-CM = 2 percent
	Virtual elimination of state mental hospitals		
By 2000			
"Teleprescriptions" commonly used	Moderate chemical control of senility	Pharmacists primarily trained for research careers	World population: 6 billion
Wrist watch TV commonly available	Effective transplantation of all organ systems except for CNS	Establishment of many CHSs	First clinic or hospital on the moon
Wide availability of computers that "learn" from experience	Development of electronic sensors enabling blind people to "see"	Robots with sensory feedback performing routine household chores in hospitals	Periodic polling of public on health care issues by computer
Full wall-sized color 3D IATV	Laboratory demonstration of regeneration or repair of destroyed neurons		P-CM = 5 percent
			H-TM = 91 percent
			M-CM = 4 percent

TABLE 3 (Continued)

Year	Communication and Computer Technology	Biomedicine and Theraputics	Education and Occupations	Miscellaneous
By 2005	Wide use of "pharmaceutical automats"	Demonstration of way to decrease time between birth and maturity Development of drugs from substances originating on other planets or the moon Human parthenogenesis	15 percent of medical schools devoted totally to training medics	P-CM = 2 percent H-TM = 88 percent M-CM = 10 percent
By 2010	Automatic reprogramming of medical computers Wide use of IATV and phonovision for psychotherapy, greatly diminishing need for outpatient psychiatric clinics	Wide use of artificial insemination to produce genetically superior offspring Use of highly complex chemical simulation models of the human body for use in drug experimentation *In vivo* renewal of worn-out hearts by stimulating natural growth processes Most forms of mental retardation are cured	Virtual cessation of pharmacy schools Reliable tests available to predict interpersonal skills of medics which are used as admission criteria Surgeons generally trained in SMIs	Breeding of new animals and plants to alter man's ecosystem for his benefit P-CM = 1 percent H-TM = 79 percent M-CM = 20 percent

By 2015	Demonstration of man-machine symbiosis, enabling people to extend their intelligence by direct electromechanical interaction between his brain and a computer "Telemedicine" services widely delivered in homes	Use of drugs or altered prenatal conditions to raise IQ of normal individuals by 10 to 20 points Laboratory demonstration of biochemical processes that stimulate growth of new organs and limbs Extrauterine development of human fetus Replacement of human organs with those derived from specially bred animals	Virtual obsolescence of the pharmacist Virtual cessation of MDs providing clinical services except for surgery	AMA disbanded Average US life expectancy 95 years old with commensurate prolongation of vigor Effective weather control thereby enhancing global food production P-CM = 1 percent H-TM = 59 percent M-CM = 40 percent
By 2020	Nationwide automated continuous clinical feedback to allow for perpetual updating of computer-rendered medical decisions 95 percent of population has medical records stored in NMDB	Electrical control of mood disorders available Demonstration of long-duration human hibernation; allows for prolonged space travel Moderate use of genetic engineering in humans by chemical substitution of DNA chains	Enormous expansion of medic training programs Virtual cessation of PA and professional nurse training programs	Wide use of self-contained dwellings using life support systems that recycle water and air to provide independence from external environment 5000 hospitals in US P-CM = 0 percent H-TM = 25 percent M-CM = 75 percent

TABLE 3 (Continued)

Year	Communication and Computer Technology	Biomedicine and Therapeutics	Education and Occupations	Miscellaneous
By 2025	Inexpensive high-capacity worldwide, regional, and local (home, hospital, business) communication (using satelites, lasers, light pipes, etc.)	Development of man-machine chimeras *In utero* genetic modification First subject using cryogenic preservation "unfrozen" without success Maintenance of human brain extracorporeally for one month	Frequent international health care seminars conducted via IATV and COMSAT	Researchers rather than surgeons (MDs) conduct most operations P-CM = 0 percent H-TM = 10 percent M-CM = 90 percent

NOTES

1. Kahn, H., and A. J. Wiener (1967). *Toward the Year 2000: A Framework for Speculation.* New York: Macmillan.

2. Baran, P. (1973). "30 Services That Two-Way Television Can Provide." *The Futurist,* 7:202–210.

3. Gabor, D. (1970). *Innovations: Scientific, Technological, and Social.* New York: Oxford University Press.

4. Bender, A. D., A. E. Strack, G. W. Ebright, and G. V. Haunalter (1969). "Delphic Study Examines Developments in Medicine." *Futures,* 1:289–303.

5. Syntheses of Phases 1 and 2 of the Delphi Enquiry into Health and the Practice of Medicine in 1980–1990. (1972). Basle, Switzerland, September 13–15.

6. Gordon, T. J., and R. H. Ament (1969). *Forecasts of Some Technological and Scientific Developments and Their Societal Consequences.* Middletown, Conn.: Institute for the Future. Number R-6.

7. McLaughlin, C. P., and A. Sheldon (1974). *The Future and Medical Care: A Health Manager's Guide to Forecasting.* Cambridge, Mass: Ballinger.

8. Maxmen, J. S. (1975). "Forecasting and Medical Education." *Journal of Medical Education,* 50:54–65.

INDEX